Operation Room Assistant Manual

Operation Room Assistant Manual

TS Jayalakshmi

Professor of Anaesthesiology
All India Institute of Medical Sciences
New Delhi-110 022

Foreword by

VA Punnoose

PEEPEE

PUBLISHERS and DISTRIBUTORS (P) LTD.

Operation Room Assistant Manual

Published by
Pawaninder P. Vij

Peepee Publishers and Distributors (P) Ltd.
Head Office: 160, Shakti Vihar, Pitam Pura
Delhi-110 034 (India)

Correspondence Address:
7/31, First Floor, Ansari Road, Daryaganj
Post Box-7243
New Delhi-110 002 (India)

Ph: 65195868, 9811156083, 23246245

e-mail: peepee160@yahoo.co.in

e-mail: peepee160@rediffmail.com

e-mail: peepee160@gmail.com

www.peepeepub.com

First Edition: **2005**
Reprint 2008
Reprint 2010

ISBN: 81-88867-47-0

Printed at
Lordson, C-5/19, Rana Pratap Bagh, Delhi-110 007

Foreword

It is heartening to see that the long-cherished desire of a great teacher and visionary has taken shape in this "Operation Room Assistant Manual". While Prof Jayalakshmi could have written books for physician-anaesthesiologists, she foresaw the great need of a practical manual to educate the non-medical staff working with anaesthesiologists and playing a vital role in patient-management during the crucial intra-operative phase. Few physicians hitherto ventured into this arena of educating the technical staff.

In the foregoing pages, one can see how the author, out of long stay in OTs, has realised the areas where an ORA need training. Rather than opting for high-profile theoretical discourse, Prof Jayalakshmi, chose to identify and stress areas in the perspective of an ORA in the OT, as a technical assistant.

Procedures are clearly explained, pharmacologic actions of all essential agents used in OT are clarified, precautions and possible complications given due place, equipment functions are explained with sketches drawn to perfection. The illustrations are brilliant. Current trends in waste disposal protocol, infection control measures, cardiopulmonary resuscitation are presented intelligibly, thanks the long experience of the author as a consummate teacher and sound clinician anaesthetist. Essentials which every ORA/OT technician must know, such as surgical positions, care of body parts of the unconscious patient, practical aspects of infection control, decontamination and biomedical waste handling are vividly explained. Section on CPR is most valuable to any OT personnel. This manual will be an indispensable companion to every ORA/OT technician in this country.

Emerit Prof: VA Punnoose
Dean of PG Studies, St Stephen Hospital
and Former Head, Cardiothorac: Anaesthesia
AIIMS, New Delhi

Preface

This is a practical operation room assistant's manual and not a textbook. No attempt is made to have a full discourse on body physiology, anatomy or pathology of disease processes.

In modern operation theatre Nurses, Operation Room Assistants (ORA), qualified Anaesthesiologists and Surgeons form an integral team. The Operation Room Assistant, plays a major role and often faces various techniques, procedures, therapeutic agents, manoeuvres, monitoring devices, resuscitation and equipments. In many hospitals, there is no formal curriculum training course for ORAs. Hence today ORAs are a silent witnesses to the routine in operation theatre and rise and gain experience mostly by observation.

This manual aims at filling the gap on the practical side of the operation room and it fulfills the natural ambition of this group to understand more on these aspects so that the contribution can be more powerful and effective. It is also intended to act as a reference guide for people guiding, teaching and training the ORAs.

The author feels that the objective would be achieved, if a new entrant gains rapid insight into the mysteries of a working day OT thereby enabling valuable, efficient service to the patient and proper back up to the operation theatre team.

My senior colleagues and teachers, Dr VA Punnoose and Dr HL Kaul have encouraged me not only to get a deep insight into various aspects but also encouraged me to improve and act on existing methodologies on various aspects. My heartfelt thanks to them.

TS Jayalakshmi

Abbreviations

ICU	Intensive Care Unit
ORA	Operation Room Assistant
OT	Operation Theatre
CSR	Central Sterilization Room
CSSD	Central Sterile Supply Department
FGF	Fresh Gas Flow
FM	Face Mask
CT	Corrugated Tube
EV	Expiratory Valve
CVP	Central Venous Pressure
HCW	Health Care Worker
VF	Ventricular Fibrillation
VT	Ventricular Tachycardia
CPR	Cardio Pulmonary Resuscitation
BMWM	Biomedical Waste Management
ETO	Ethylene Oxide

Contents

1

Anaesthesia Technician and Operation Room Assistant (ORA)

The anaesthesia assistant or operating room assistant (ORA) must familiarize himself/herself with the basic principles of all the anaesthetic gadgets, theatre installations and drugs used in the theatres in which she/he works.

- It is the anaesthetist's direct responsibility to ensure that the equipments are in good working order before use. He may entrust some of such duties to the ORA.
- The anaesthesia assistant or ORA having basic knowledge on the utility of the equipment may obtain further information from the manufacturer's brochure supplied with such anaesthesia/theatre equipment, and from anaesthesiologist.
- Information about new machines and equipments obtained from the technical booklets supplied along with particular machine, has to be clearly understood before putting it to use.
- The servicing and maintenance of anaesthetic equipments, accessories and monitors is the task of the hospital's maintenance unit. Procurement of machines and accessories is the duty of the administration.
- Information regarding the functions, handling, safety precautions, the do's and dont's are important for the safety of patients and longevity of the equipment.
- The ORA should make a mandatory check of the working status of each equipment, every morning.

- He also shall keep the appropriate accessories and drugs required for the specific procedure, before the start, under instruction from anaesthetist.
- He should also ensure that all consumables used up are duly replaced and stored in appropriate places. Every item in theatre must have a specific place, well known to all those working in O.T., so that they can be easily brought out in a crisis.

What is Expected of a Technician in the O.T.?

- Safe keeping of equipments.
- Periodic checking for faults, care of gas cylinders, suction units.
- Daily laying out of them for routine use.
- Collection, cleaning and return to safe storage place.
- Cleaning and Carbolising anaesthesia machine and monitors daily before start of anaesthesia.
- Equipment/pieces/parts requiring other forms of sterilization to be carried out: e.g. Formaldehyde preservation, cidex treatment, E.T.O. sterilization. He should have clear knowledge on these procedures.
- Proficiency in handling things with asceptic precautions.
- Familiarity with infusion pumps, arterial lines, transducers, 3-ways, central lines, fibre optic equipments and care of handling them.
- Methods of sterilization.
- Common pathogens in OT's and ICU's.
- Familiarity with all infusions, their indication, care of handling infusions and transfusions.
- Packing of items such as spinal sets, injection trays and forward them for C.S.R daily or if possible get them sterilized in OT complex.
- Keep account of stocks and stores of perishable, consumable items and for scheduled drugs.
- Understand the requisition of each operation/ anaesthesia and keep such things ready before start of anaesthetic circuits, LMA, scavenging, disposables.

- Legal and moral aspects of proper check on blood-transfusion.
- Drill in emergency care: Air embolism, drug anaphylaxis, intra arterial thiopentone, local anaesthetic toxicity, convulsions, acute severe bleeding, malignant hyperpyrexia, cardiac arrest.
- How to assist anaesthetist without interferring.
- Methodology and system in handling things.
- Aseptic care.
- Ordering for blood and blood-products from blood-bank, cross-checking the details on labels.
- Tidiness in laying the anaesthesia machines/trolley with syringe tray, BP, laryngoscope, airways, swabs etc. used items each in its proper place according to ISO directives.
- Familiar with setting up monitors—Pulse oximetry, capnograph, ECG, transducers, pressure monitors and lines, infusion-pumps, defibrillators, chest-drain systems, CVP system, sources of technical errors, blood-loss monitors, paediatric canopy, warming mattress, temperature monitors, over-head lights, TV/video installation.
- Should get experience in the requirements specific to different types of surgery, operating postures, care of pressure-points, and use of fibre-optic devices.
- Should have basic knowledge of diseases, such as diabetes, hypertension, bronchial asthma, renal, hepatic diseases, coronary disease, anaemias, and endocrine disorders, of full-term pregnancy. Caesarean section, and resuscitation of neonate.
- Should be aware of complications possible in each surgical and anaesthetic procedures, acid-base, electrolyte disturbances, arrhythmias, bronchospasm during operation and at recovery.

2

Anaesthesia Room

- The anaesthesia room is meant for intravenous access, induction of general anaesthesia, performance of regional techniques, monitoring and to keep patient calm.
- The anaesthesia room should have a tiltable and movable table, anaesthesia machine, intubation equipments, drug trolley, noninvasive blood pressure and oxygen saturation monitoring equipments and a suction apparatus, assortment of tracheal tubes, canula, drugs and infusions.
- Some hospitals may not utilise this room, and anaesthetic procedures are carried out inside O.R. However, the setting can be alarming to the patient.

3

Anaesthesia: General Principles

Anaesthesia can be:

a. General
b. Spinal, subarchnoid/epidural
c. Regional nerve(s) block.

Consciousness is lost in the first, but not in (b) and (c). General anaesthesia is achieved by intravenous or inhalational routes of administration.

The sequence of events are, premedication, induction, maintenance, and recovery.

- Patient receives a combination of drugs before induction of anaesthesia which is called premedication meant to make the patient tranquil and drowsy, suppress vagal reflexes, reduce gastric acid, and inhibit secretions.
- The first step to general anaesthesia is induction which can be achieved by administration of intravenous drugs or inhalational agents.
- Once the patient is induced, or put to sleep, further unconciousness and adequate analgesia for surgical procedures will be maintained by continued administration of anaesthetic gases/ vapors or by intravenous injection/infusion of one or more other drugs.
- At the end of surgery, the patient is reverted to his conscious level often by termination of anaesthetic administration, and where necessary, by relevant antagonist drugs.

4

Gases Used in Anaesthesia

OXYGEN (O_2)

Oxygen (O_2) essential gas used for life support during anaesthesia.

- Oxygen is colourless and odourless gas and is stored in metal cylinders at very high pressure (2000 PSI or 132 atmosphere).
- Where oxygen consumption is more than 150,000 litres per week usually, piped oxygen is used from a bank of oxygen cylinders (called manifold) ensuring a continuous supply (Fig. 4.1). Liquid oxygen store is also used where consumption is very large and is economical.

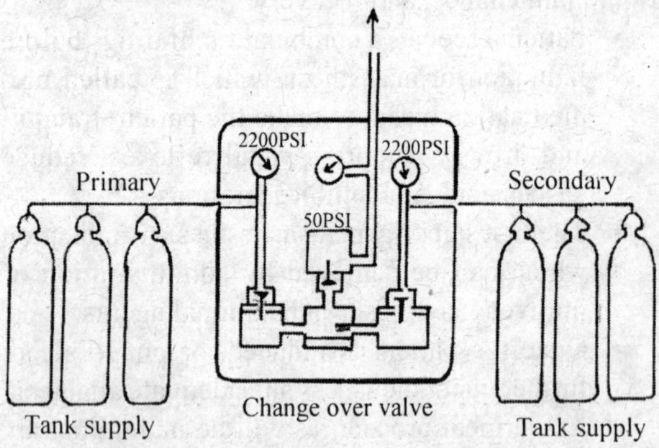

Fig. 4.1: Simplified version of pipeline supply from a manifold room

- The cylinder is coloured black with white shoulder (top). In some countries (US), it is all green.
- Oxygen concentrators are useful both in hospitals and in long term domicillary oxygen therapy where oxygen is produced from ambient air.

- It is used as an essential carrier gas during general anaesthesia, along with nitrous oxide, and one of the anaesthetic vapours.
- O_2 is given as a supplementation in sick, elderly, hypoxic, high risk patients in shock, and gas poisoning.
- During prolonged oxygen therapy and in infants humidified oxygen is mandatory.
- The oxygen cylinder supply should be assessed both before and during anaesthesia.
- The empty cylinder is changed promptly after opening the stand-by cylinder first outside O.R., and then at the time of use.
- Cylinder key to be kept in the machine for ready use.
- Flush type cylinder is opened by using cylinder valve handles (key) (Fig. 4.2).

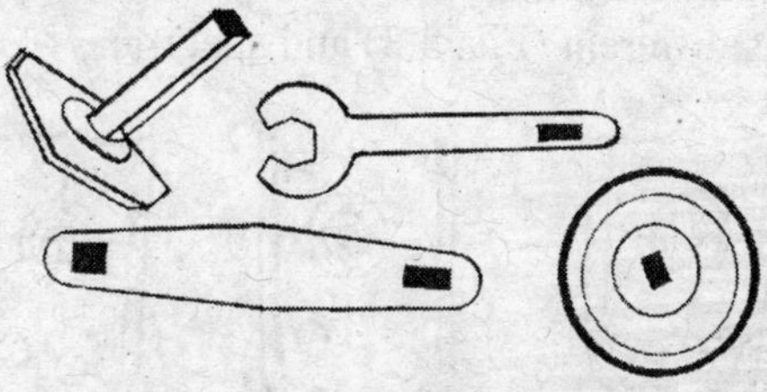

Fig. 4.2: Flush type cylinder valve handles (key) for opening the cylinder. ■ = Indicates holes in the key which fits into the cylinder valve. For Bull-nose type cylinder valve, wrench is used to open the cylinder

- The duration of use of an oxygen cylinder time depends on the flow of oxygen and the size of cylinder used.
- Due allowance should be given to wastage due to flushing of circuits by high flows periodically and to possible leakage.

Oxygen cylinders

Type	*Capacity (L)*
A	76
B	196
C	396

Contd...

Contd...

Type	*Capacity (L)*
D	659
E	2062
F	3000
G	5321
H and K	5570

C and D are used on anaesthesia machines.

SAFETY PRECAUTIONS INCORPORATED IN OXYGEN CYLINDERS

- To avoid wrong cylinder connection to anaesthesia machine, non-interchangeable flush type (pin-index) valves are used. The outlet valves of flush type cylinders have two holes in the positions which will fit on to the corresponding pins on the yolk of the machine. The position of holes for each gas is different (Fig. 4.3) and specific.

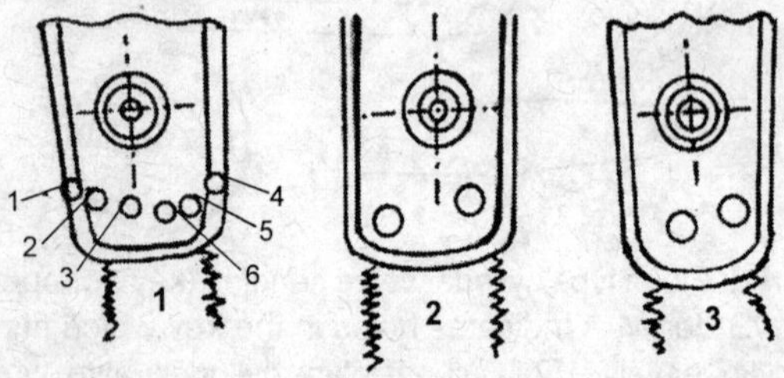

Fig. 4.3: Various positions of holes in Flush-type cylinder outlet. (1=Master index; 2=Oxygen 2,5; 3=Nitrous oxide 3,5)

NITROUS OXIDE (N_2O)

This is an anaesthetic gas, the other being cyclopropane which is not widely used. This gas is stored in blue cylinders as a liquid at a pressure of 50 bar (750 1b/sq inch). The gas also can be provided through a pipe line from a manifold room. This cylinder should be kept vertical during use so that the liquid phase remains at the bottom and the gas above the liquid is delivered to the patient. N_2O is a sweet smelling, non-irritant, colourless gas and it is not inflammable but supports combustion of fuels in the absence of oxygen.

IMPORTANT PROPERTIES

1. It is a good analgesic but weak anaesthetic.
2. It is essential to administer a minimum of 30% oxygen while giving N_2O and it should not be used as a sole anaesthetic agent, as it lacks adequate potency for surgery.
3. It can be used with other inhalational agents.
4. At the termination of anaesthesia 100% oxygen should be administered to flush out all the gas and to avoid diffusion hypoxia.
5. It may not be used in one lung anaesthesia, laser surgery, high altitudes, closed body cavities filled with air, in hypoxic states, and if air–embolism is suspected.

A reserve cylinder should always be kept ready. Various types and capacities of Nitrous oxide cylinder available are given below:

Nitrous Oxide Gas Cylinders

Type	*Capacity (L)*
A	189
B	378
*C	946
*D	1,590
E	5,260
F	7,570
G	13,836
H and K	15,899

* C and D are commonly used on anaesthesia machines

5

Inhalational Anaesthetic Agents

Volatile Inhalational Anaesthetic Agents

- These are liquids, vaporized at ambient temperatures, in containers called either vaporizers or inhalers.
- These inhalational agents can be classified as:

  A. Agents of historical interest:
  Ethyl chloride
  Divinyl ether
  Choloroform
  Methoxyflurane

  B. Agents occasionally used:
  Diethyl ether
  Trichloroethylene

  C. Agents commonly used:
  i. Halothane
  Isoflurane
  Enflurane
  ii. Desflurane, Sevoflurane } newer agents

Ethylene, cyclopropane and nitrous oxide are compressed anaesthetic gases, in cylinders.

Diethyl Ether

This agent is still used in developing countries like India and other third world countries. It is inexpensive and has a wide margin of safety. It is inflammable and should not be used in the presence of surgical cautery, or open flame. The agent can be used by inhalers like ether bottle, and by calibrated vaporizers (ethertec, 'Vapor' vaporizer, EMO) (Figs 5.1 to 5.3b).

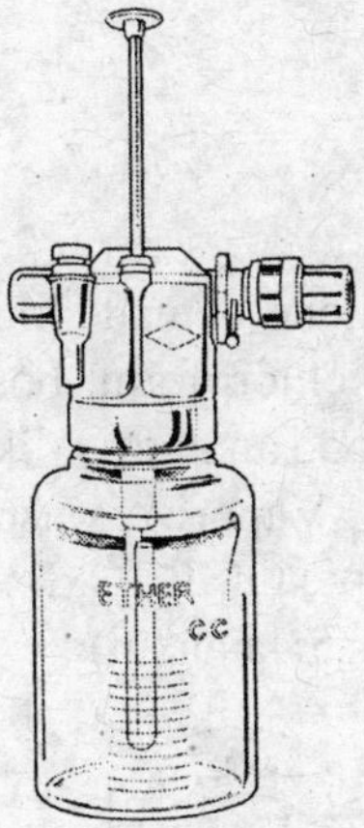

Fig. 5.1: Boyle's bottle

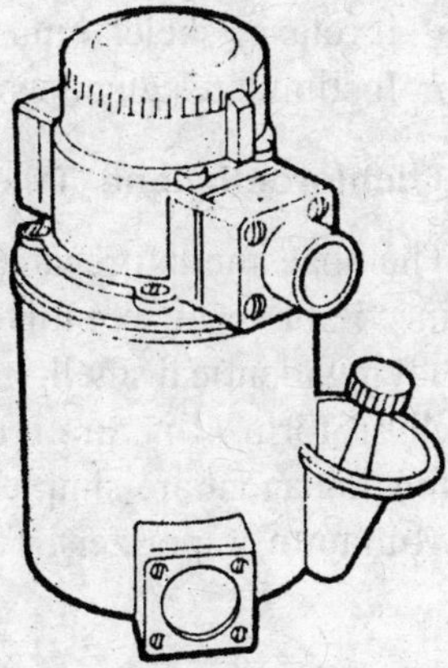

Fig. 5.2: Screw cap filler for Diethyl-Ether

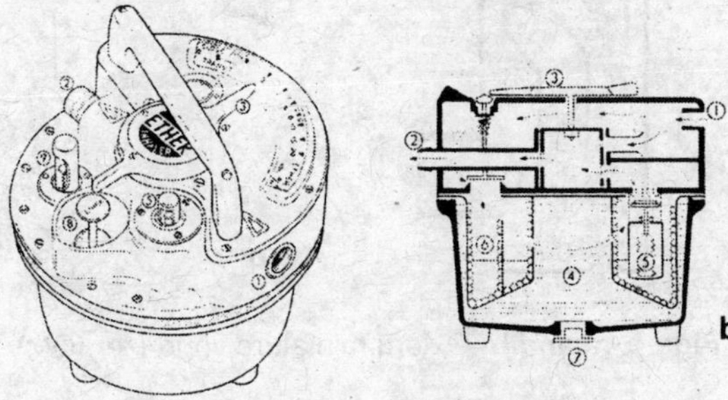

a b

Figs 5.3a and b: EMO vaporizer

It can be safely used with a closed circuit, with sodalime.

A closed circuit is a gas saving breathing system where expired gas from patient is re-used. Its CO_2 is then absorbed by passing the gases through sodalime.

Peculiarities of Ether are that

- It is irritant to respiratory tract, has a pungent smell.
- Deep planes produces bronchial muscle relaxation.
- It increases the salivary and bronchial secretion.
- Post operative nausea and vomiting are occasionally seen.
- Infiltration of local anaesthetics with adrenaline is safe with ether anaesthesia. (Unlike with halogenated hydrocarbons like halothane).

- It relaxes skeletal muscles.
- It stimulates gluconeogenesis.

Trichloroethylene (Trilene)

The anaesthetic preparation of trilene is made blue in colour to differentiate it from chloroform, both having identical smell. It is very good analgesic, like chloroform, it is rarely used now. Vaporizers used for this agent are simple bottle type, OMC (Oxford Miniature Vaporizer), Tritec (Figs 5.4a and b).

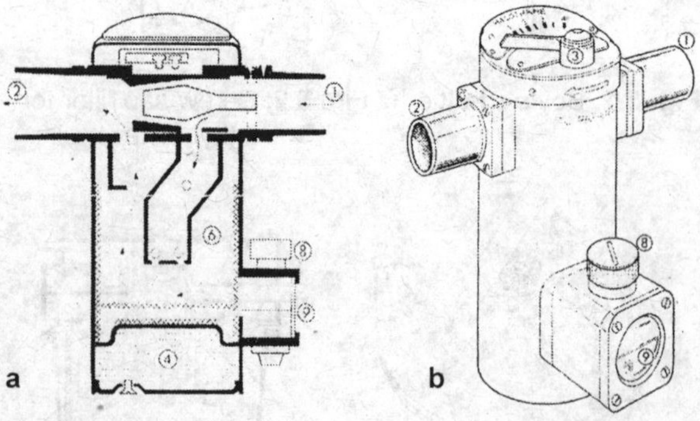

Figs 5.4a and b: Oxford miniature vaporizer (OMV)

Important Properties

- Has powerful analgesic effect.
- It does not produce any skeletal muscle relaxation.
- This agent should not be used along with sodalime. At temperature above 50°C it produces toxic $COCl_2$ (phosgene).
- This agent can be used for obstetric patients for analgesia.
- Cardiac arrythmias are likely with this drug in presence of endogenous or exogenous catecholamines (infiltration of local anaesthetic with adrenaline or adrenaline pack).
- Recovery is delayed with this agent.

Halothane

It is a colourless liquid, non-inflammable, and is the most widely used agent, the world over today.

Vaporizers used for halothane are—Goldman and 'Tec' type vaporizers (Figs 5.5a to c).

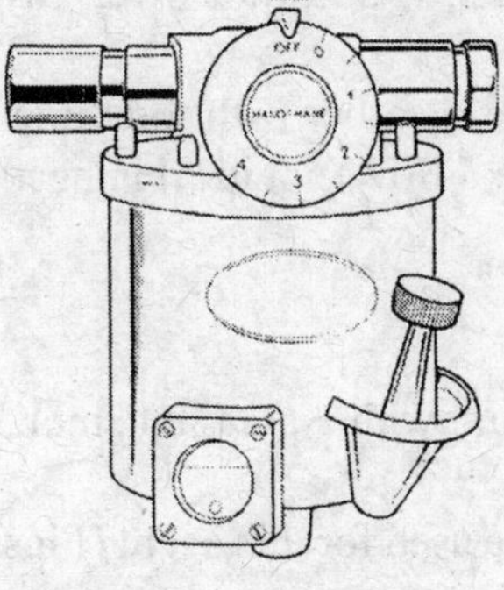

Fig. 5.5a: Fluotec Mk II

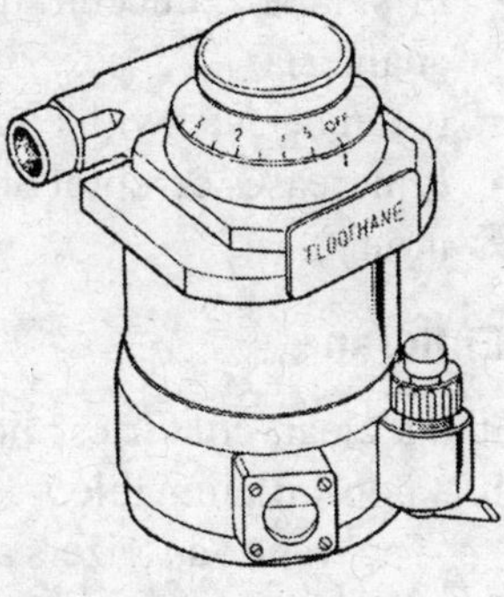

Fig. 5.5b: Fluotec Mk III

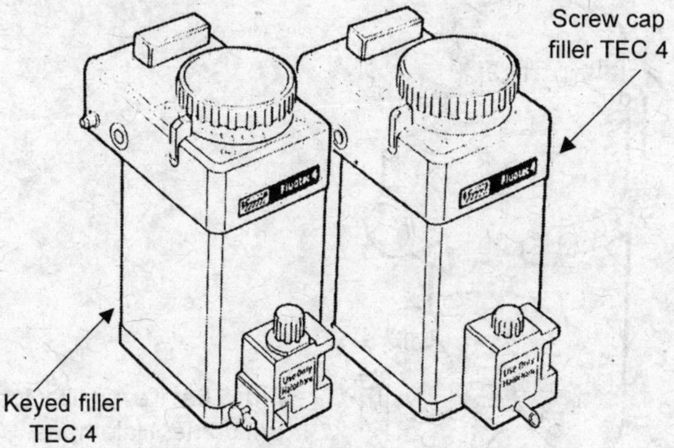

Fig. 5.5c: Keyed filler and screw cap filler

Important Properties

- Non-irritant to breathe, produce bronchodilation. Rapid loss of pharyngeal and laryngeal reflexes and inhibition of salivary and bronchial secretions.
- Halothane is a potent myocardial depressant which is dose related.
- Cardiac arrythmias may occur during halothane anaesthesia. It sensitizes the myocardium to endogeneous and exogeneous catecholamines.
- Post operative nausea and vomiting are minimal.
- It relaxes the uterine and skeletal muscles.
- On rare occasions halothane may be associated with the production of hepatic dysfunction.

- It produces rapid and smooth induction and relatively a rapid recovery.
- In smaller concentrations, it does not offer any analgesia.
- It can be used with circle absorber with sodalime.
- It increases cerebral blood flow (not ideal in head injury).

Enflurane

It is a clear, colourless liquid with a pleasant smell. It is non-inflammable.

'Tec' type vaporizers are used for this agent (Figs 5.6a and b).

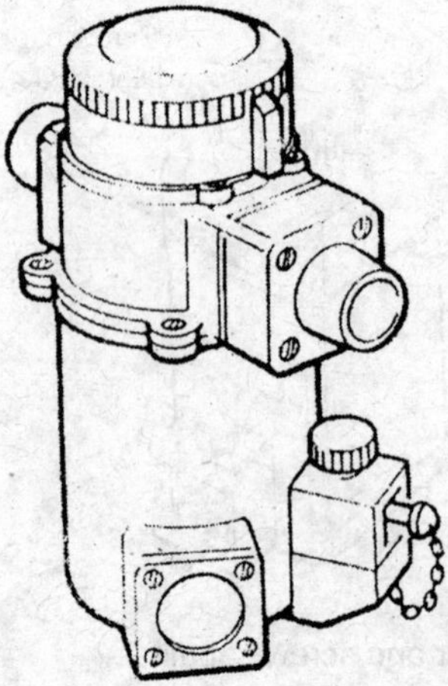

Fig. 5.6a: Keyed filler for Enflurane, Halothane

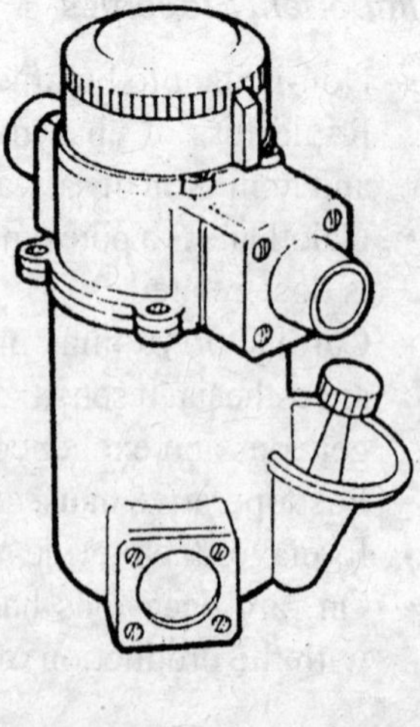

Fig. 5.6b: Screw cap filler for Enflurane, Halothane, Trichoroethylene

Important Properties

- Rapid induction and recovery.
- Non irritant to respiratory tract and do not increase secretions.
- Dose dependant myocardial depression with smaller incidence of arrhythmias than halothane and less sensitisation of myocardium to catecholamines, either endogenous or exogenous.
- It relaxes uterine muscle which is dose dependant.
- It produces epileptiform paroxysmal spine activity and burst suppression. To be avoided in epileptics.
- It produces skeletal muscle relaxation and potentiates muscle relaxants.
- It can be used with sodalime absorber.
- Risk of renal and hepatotoxicity very minimal.
- The main disadvantage is its high cost and occasional seizure activity on EEG.

Isoflurane

It is a colourless, volatile liquid with rather pungent odour. 'Tec' tupe vaporizer is used for this agent.

Important Properties

- Rapid induction and recovery.
- Myocardial depressant effect very minimal and dose dependant.
- Produces bronchodilatation and relaxation of uterine muscle.
- Produces skeletal muscle relaxation and protentiates muscle relaxants (like Halothane).
- Seizure activity on EEG is absent (unlike Enflurane).
- It can be used with sodalime with circle absorber (unlike Trilene).
- The main disadvantages are high cost, pungent odour, coronary vasodilatation.

6

Intravenous Anaesthetic Agents

Intravenous (IV) anaesthetic agents are used commonly to induce anaesthesia. It is more rapid and smoother compared with inhalational agents. These agents can be used for maintenance of anaesthesia by continuous infusion. They are classified as:

A. Rapidly acting agents:
   1. Thiopentone, Methohexitone (Barbiturate)
   2. Etomidate (Imidozole compound)
   3. Propofol (Phenol group)
   4. Propanidid (Eugenol derivative, no longer in use)
   5. Althesin (Steroid, no longer in use)
   6. Midazolam (Benzodiazepine).

B. Slower acting:
   1. Ketamine (Phencyclidine derivative)
   2. Diazepam (Benzodiazepine derivative).
   3. Morphine, Fentanyl, Alfentanyl, Sufentanyl (Opioids)
   4. Haloperidol, Droperidol (Butyrophenone).

THIOPENTONE SODIUM: (PENTOTHAL, INTRAVAL)

It is a yellow powder and is soluble in distilled water, 2.5% solution is preferred for intravenous injection (1 gm in 40 mls). In solution it is not very stable, beyond 24 hours unless refrigerated. The solution can be used safely provided it is clear. It is supplied in ampoules and multi-dose vials. Average dose required is 3-5 mg/kg body weight intravenously for induction.

Uses

It is used as an induction agent, as an infusion to control convulsive states and as anaesthetic for modified electroconvulsive therapy. Anaesthesia with thiopentone should never be undertaken lightly. Resuscitation trolley, oxygen source, a short acting relaxant, intubation set, and intravenous line are all to be kept ready before the administration of drug.

PROPOFOL

It is extremely lipid soluble but insoluble in water. Ampoules of the drug contain 200 mg of propofol in 20 ml (10 mg/ml). Loss of verbal contact is used as end point during propofol induction, (for thiopentone the equivalent as disappearance of eyelash reflex). A dose of 2-2.5 mg/kg is required to induce anaesthesia in healthy unpremedicated adults.

Uses

This drug is used for induction of anaesthesia, sedation during surgery, total intravenous anaesthesia and for sedation in intensive care units. It is more suitable than thiopentone for outpatient anaesthesia because of rapid early recovery of conciousness.

KETAMINE HYDROCHLORIDE

It produces dissociative anaesthesia rather than generalized central nervous system depression. It is soluble in water and is presented as solutions of 10 mg/ml, 50 mg/ml or 100 mg/ml in multidose vials. It is a very good analgesic and it can be used intravenously as well as intramuscularly. The IV dose is 2 mg/kg and IM dose is 8 mg/kg body weight.

Its main disadvantages are emergence delirium, night-mares and hallucinations which can be obviated by pre-medicating the patients with benzodiazepines. It also produces tachycardia, hypertension, salivation and raised intracranial and intraocular pressure.

Uses

It is used as an induction agent in patients in shock being resusciated by fluids or blood and in paediatrics outdoor patients for minor surgical procedures. It is very useful at outdoor sites of accidents and in field conditions where anaesthesia is required.

MORPHINE SULPHATE

Morphine is a narcotic analgesic.

- It supresses awareness, anxiety, pain sensation and respiration.
- It produces broncho-constriction and billiary spasm.
- It can cause nausea and vomiting.
- It does not disturb cardiovascular functions.

Uses

It is used as a pre-medicant, and as an induction agent in shock patients and cardiac cases, and analgesic supplement during general anaesthesia, and in post-operative analgesia (by intra-muscular, intravenous, subarachnoid or epidural route). It is also used for patient–controlled analgesia (PCA) where a patient can administer analgesia in small doses as and when required through a special syringe pump.

FENTANYL, ALFENTANYL, SUFENTANYL

All these are potent, short acting narcotics. Their properties are similar to morphine. Since these are short acting, they are used commonly for induction purposes, and continuous infusion.

DIAZEPAM

This is a minor tranquilliser, and amnesic

- It is insoluble in water, and precipitates with many anaesthetic drugs.
- IV injection is painful.
- It is also used as an induction agent in poor risk patients.
- Mainly it is used as premedicant, anticonvulsant, sedative during regional techniques, for cardio-version, adjuvant to local anaesthesia during endoscopic procedures and dental surgery.

- It should not be mixed with other drugs, nor added to infusions.
- It should be injected into a large vein for fear of phlebitis.

MIDAZOLAM

This is a short acting, water soluble benzodiazepine. It is used for induction of anaesthesia.

It is available in 2 ml (5 mg ml^{-1}) ampoules. If necessary it can be diluted (diazepam cannot be diluted).

15 mg tablet also available for oral use.

Dosage for different purposes are:

- Premedication – 15 mg orally or 5 mg i.m.
- Sedation – 2-7 mg i.v., incremental bolus of 0.5-1 mg
- For status epilepticus–not recommended.

DROPERIDOL, HALOPERIDOL

Droperidol is a powerful antiemetic 2.5 mg dose intravenously is used to provide antiemesis without any sedation. It is used as an neuroleptanalgesia in combination with fentanyl.

Haloperidol is also a potent antiemetic with a high incidence of skeletal muscle rigidity. It is used in psychiatric practice and in intensive care unit for agitated patients.

Both oral and parenteral preparations are available.

7

Non-anaesthetic Drugs Used in Anaesthesia

Other drugs used during anaesthesia are:
1. Muscle relaxants.
2. Antisialogogues.
3. Anti cholinesterases.
4. Vasopressors.
5. Antihypertensives and vasodilators.
6. Resuscitation drugs.

Muscle Relaxants

They block impulse transmissions at neuro-muscular junction. They are of two types:

a. Depolarisers–e.g. suxamethonium (Scoline)

b. Non-depolarisers–e.g.
   Gallamine, Tubocurare
   Pancuronium (Pavulon)
   Alcuronium
   Atracurium
   Vecuronium
   Mivacurium
   Doxacurium
   Pipecuronium

- They all produce skeletal muscle paralysis, including respiratory muscles.
- The muscle relaxants are used to produce muscle relaxation during intubation and anaesthesia.
- Suxamethonium is the drug commonly used for intubation of trachea.
- It does not require any drug for its reversal of effect.
- All non-depolarising muscles relaxants except atracurium require anticholinesterase drugs for its reversal of effect.

- Relaxants are chosen according to the clinical condition of the patient.
- Drugs which are excreted through the kidneys like gallamine are avoided in patients with acute and chronic renal failure.
- These relaxants are given either as intermittent doses or as slow infusion.

Anticholinesterases

Neostigmine sulphate is the commonly used anti-cholinestrase for the reversal of non-depolarising muscle relaxants at the end of operation.

- It is given along with the anti cholinergics like atropine sulphate, or glycopyrollate.
- The adequacy of neuromuscular reversal is judged clinically as well as by neuromuscular monitoring.

Antisialogogue

These produce drying of the salivary and bronchial secretions.

- The drugs include atropine sulphate, glycopyrrolate and hyoscine.
- These are used in pre-medication along with sedatives and narcotics, to reduce salivary secretions.
- Atropine is used to correct sinus bradycardia (slow pulse rate).
- It is also used along with neostigmine to block the relaxant effect.
- Hyoscine, apart from its antisialagogue action, can produce amnesia and drowsiness.

Pressor Agents

The naturally occurring pressor agents include adrenaline, noradrenaline and dopamine.They stimulate sympathetic receptors on heart, blood vessels, besides gut, liver, bronchi and muscles. They act through sympathetic alpha or beta receptors.

Adrenaline

It is a very potent vasopressor and cardiotonic catecholamine.

It produces vasoconstriction, it is used along with local anaesthetics to reduce toxicity and prolong duration of action, local infiltration with adrenaline provides skin ischaemia, there by reducing bleeding, in cardiac arrest, and resuscitation, for anaphylactic shock, and is used as a bronchodilator in severe bronchospasm.

Precautions

- Untoward actions include anxiety, tachycardia, palpitation, restlessness, throbbing headache, vertigo and high blood sugar levels. So dilute solutions should be used.
- It should be used with care when inhalational anaesthetic agents like trichloroethylene or halothane is used.
- It should be avoided in hypertensives, thyrotoxic and diabetics and those who receive tricyclic antidepressants and monoamine oxidase inhibitors (used in psychiatry)
- It *should not be used* with local analgesic in ring block of the digit or penis or of the external ear.
- The ampule of adrenaline and atropine look alike, so it is to be checked carefully before use.
- The patient should be carefully watched during the administration of any vasopressors.

Noradrenaline

This drug unlike adrenaline is used for its vasopressor effects only (alpha–adrenergic receptor stimulation).

It is used in patients in whom the peripheral vascular resistance is low-(as seen after removal of phaeochromocytoma), to increase peripheral vascular resistance and blood pressure.

Ephedrine

It has direct action on alpha and beta adrenergic receptors.

The autonomic nervous system has two components:

- Sympathetic and parasympathetic.

Sympathetic system controls heart and circulation by two different receptors:

Alpha and beta—alpha on blood-vessels, and beta on the heart and lungs.

It is used to control hypotension during spinal analgesia and to relieve bronchospasm. It is safe during halogenated inhalational anaesthesia.

Metaraminol (Aramine) and Methoxamine (Vasoxine) are Synthetic Vasopressors

They do not produce any cardiac dysrhythmias with halogenated inhalational agents like halothane or trichloroethylene.

Phenylephrine

- It is an alpha stimulator and in large doses beta-stimulator.
- Chief effect is on blood vessels and produces vasconstriction.
- It is used with local anaesthetics in place of adrenaline.
- It sensitizes the heart to catecholamines so should be careful while halothane and trichloroethylene anaesthesia.

Dopamine

It is a beta-adrenergic stimulant.

- It improves cardiac contractility without increasing the myocardial oxygen consumption.
- So it is used in cardiogenic shock to improve blood pressure.

- It increases the renal blood flow so used to improve urine output.
- Patients should be normovolemic before the use, of any drug that exerts its effect through these adrenergic receptors, on the blood vessel calibre.

Dobutamine

It is a derivative of dopamine with beta-stimulating effect.

- No specific effect on the renal vessels.
- When cardiac dysrhythmias are a problem, this is the drug of choice for improving circulation.

Isoprenaline

It improves the contraction of heart and increases the heart rate (beta effect).

- It causes severe peripheral vasodilatation–so adequate volume replacement is very essential before this drug is started.
- It is a good bronchodilator. Apart from infusion, sublingual tablets are used. It improves renal blood flow.
- It is used to treat heart blocks until a suitable pace-maker is implanted and also in cardiogenic shock, being a strong beta stimulator.

Salbutamol and Terbutaline

These are selective beta-stimulants with very little action on heart.

- They are mainly used as bronchodilators in the form of aerosol inhaler, can be used intravenously, subcutaneous or orally.

Antihypertensives and Vasodilators

To control the hypertensive responses during anaesthesia, antihypertensives and vasodilators are used. In certain surgical procedures, deliberate hypotension (induced hypotension) is advocated. This include major head and neck operations, ligation of patent ductus arteriosus, coarctation of aorta, vascular tumors and phaeochromocytoma. The drugs used to produce hypotension are sodium nitroprusside (SNP) and Nitroglycerin (NTG) infusion. Halothane or isoflurane anaesthesia, will facilitate the technique.

- For control of hypertensive responses, nifedipine is used sublingually.
- Deepening of anaesthesia sometimes help to control blood pressure.

Aminophyllin

To control bronchospasm.

Steroids

To control bronchospasm and to control allergic reactions to drugs and for patient receiving steroids recently.

- Steroids are also used in acute hypotension or shock and in laryngeal oedema.
- It is used as a replacement therapy in adrenalectomy patients.

Calcium Chloride

Calcium is used to improve myocardial contactility.

- Citrate toxicity is a complication of massive blood transfusion. To combat this calcium chloride is given. Also used in cardiac arrest, anaphylaxis, hyperkalemia, tetany.
- Sometimes to improve neuromuscular recovery.

Sodium Bicarbonate

It is an alkaline solution used to correct metabolic acidosis which is not immediately self–correcting.

Local Anaesthetic Agents

These are agents which blocks the nerve impulse conduction.

- Local anaesthetics affect not only nerve fibres but all types of excitable tissues including smooth and striated muscle.

- Local anaesthetic agents are used for different–regional techniques such as:
  a. Infiltration anaesthesia–where the local anaesthetics are injected at the site of operation (Incision).
  b. Field block–local agent injected over the operative field.
  c. Nerve block by depositing local anaesthetic agent near the big nerve or nerves supplying the area to be operated on.
  d. Topical or surface analgesia–only over the mucous membrane or cornea.
  e. Intravenous local analgesia. An extremity of the body is made numb by injecting the drug intravenously after applying a tourniquet proximally. This is Bier's technique.
  f. Subarachnoid and epidural analgesia-injecting the local anaesthetic agents in the spinal canal either in the subrachnoid space or in the epidural space.

Cocaine Hydrochloride

- It is extracted from leaves of Erythroxylum coca.
- It is a powerful vasoconstrictor.
- It is used only as a surface analgesia.
- Used as a spray to reduce nasal congestion and analgesia.
- It is a powerful central nervous system stimulant and can induce convulsions.
- The safe dose is 4% solution 2 ml.
- Duration of action 20 min.
- Very rarely used nowadays, being a drug of addiction.

Procaine Hydrochloride (Novocaine)

- It is used for nerve blocks and the strength is 0.25–1%.
- For extradural block 5% solution is used.
- It is relatively non toxic.
- Duration of action 45 to 90 min.

- It is recommended intravenously for the treatment of malignant hyperpyrexia. No longer popular due to anaphylaxis.

Lignocaine Hydrochloride (Xylocaine)

- Most commonly used local analgesic agent.
- For infiltration 0.25% to 0.5% is used with adrenaline 1-250, 000.
- 4% is used for topical analgesia.
- For nerve block 1.5% to 2% with or without ardenaline.
- Extradural block 1 to 2% with or without ardenaline.
- For topical surface analgesia for cornea 4% solution is used.
- 1-2% jelly is used for urethral analgesia, lubricating endotracheal and nasogastric tubes.
- 2% viscous is used for throat analgesia.
- For subarachnoid block–5% solution was used.
- The recommended dose with adrenaline is 5-7 mg per kilogram body weight (maximum 500 mg) and without adrenaline 3 mg/kg body weight not exceeding 200 mg.
- Duration of action shorter(1 to 2 hrs).
- The toxic effects are twitching, convulsion, respiratory depression and acute cardiac failure.
- Plain xylocaine without preservative intravenously is used for venticular arrhythmias.

Precaution

- Local anaesthetics with adrenaline should not be used for infiltration of penis, tip of nose, fingers or pinna of ear since it produces severe vasconstriction leading to ischaemia and gangrene, and should be avoided in cardiac and hypertensive patients.

Bupivacaine (Marcaine)

This drug is also used commonly. It is a long acting local anaesthetic agent.

- It is more potent than lignocaine.

- It is a cardiotoxic agent and should not be **used intravenously.**
- Duration of action prolonged (5 hrs.)
- The safe dose is 0.2 mg/kg body weight for subarachnoid block.
- Strength used is 0.125–0.75 % with or without adrenaline.
- It is used for infiltration analgesia, extradural block, and subarachnoid block.

Other Local Anaesthetic Agents

Include Chloroprocaine, Amethocaine, Mepivacaine, Etidocaine, Prilocaine and Cinchocaine which are not used commonly in India.

8

Anaesthesia Equipment and Breathing Circuits

This includes:

A. Anaesthesia delivery systems
   1. Anaesthesia Machine, Breathing circuits and intubation sets (airway management equipments).
   2. Ventilator.

B. Instrumentation
   1. Monitoring anaesthesia delivery system. (Equipment Monitors).
   2. Monitoring the patient (Patient Monitors).

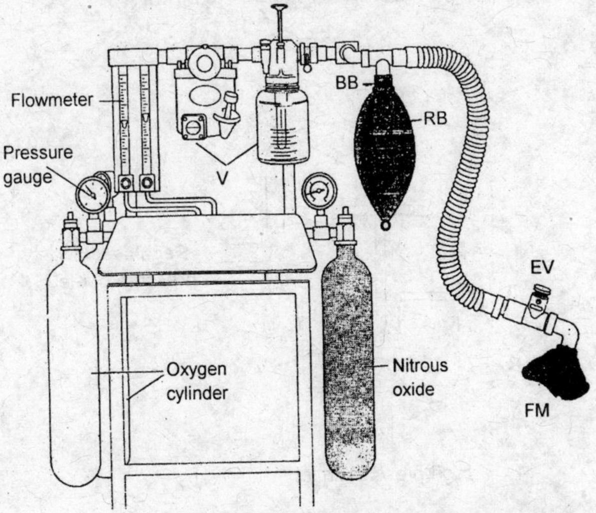

V = Vaporizer; RB = Reservior bag; EV = Expiratory valve; FM = Face mask; BB = Boyle bottle

Fig. 8.1: Anaesthesia machine with Magills circuit. Basic Anaesthesia Machine

Basic Anaesthesia Machine

Supply of Gases

- These are designed to use gases from pipeline of a manifold room, or from cylinder's (O_2 N_2O and air).
- These high pressure compressed gases are delivered to patients after duly reducing the pressure by using reducing valves (Regulator) (Figs 8.2a and b).

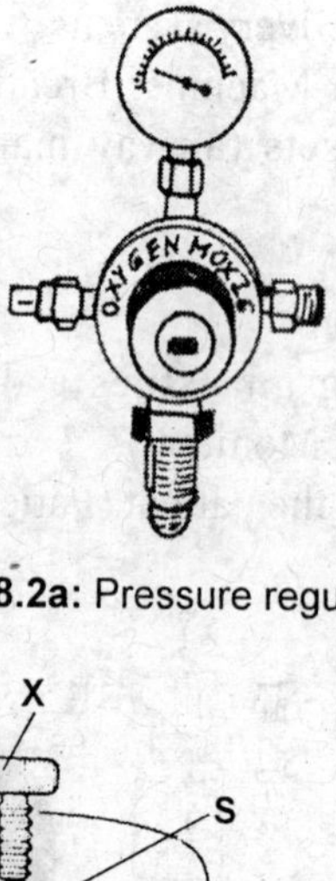

Fig. 8.2a: Pressure regulator

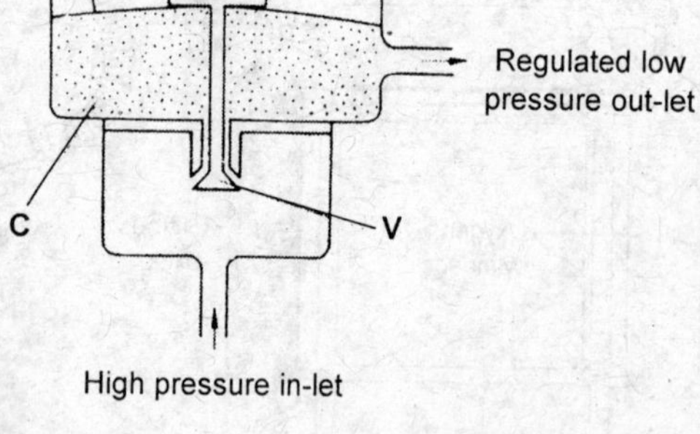

S = spring; C = low pressure; V = valve seating; D = diaphragm; X = adjustment screw

Fig. 8.2b: Cross section-pressure regulator—A simple pressure regulator-cross section showing important parts

- The content pressure in the cylinder is reflected in the pressure gauge attached to the cylinder (Fig. 8.3).

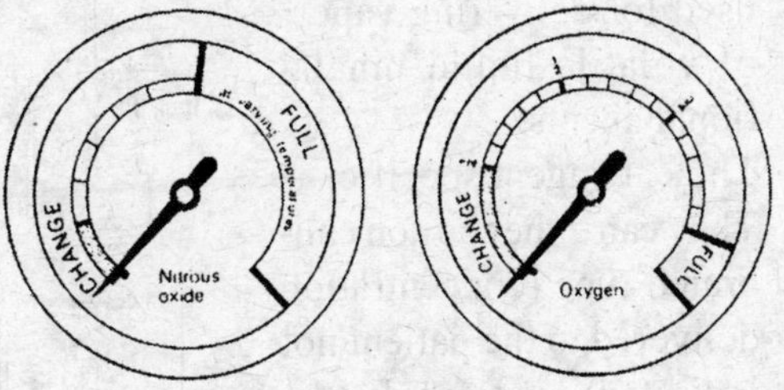

Fig. 8.3: Nitrous oxide and oxygen cylinder contents gauges

Flowmeters

- After pressure reduction, the gases pass through 'flowmeters' which are built in anesthesia machine (Fig. 8.4).

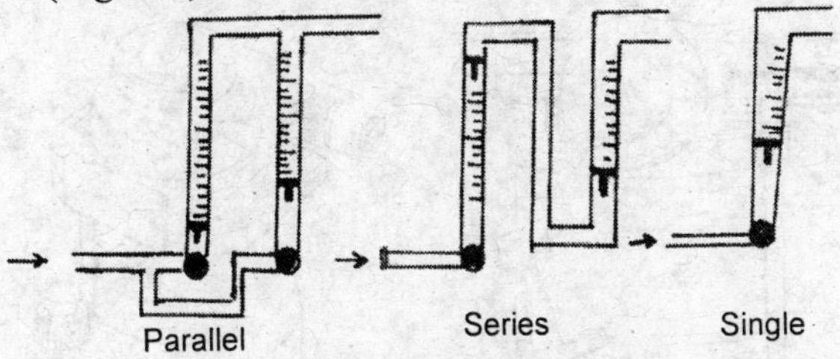

(→ = Fresh gas flone; **T** = Bobbin (Float); ● = Control knob

Fig. 8.4: Flowmeter arrangements in different anaesthesia machines

- Flowmeters are calibrated for accurate gas supply.
- They are arranged in parallel, series or single.
- It consists of a needle valve and a rotameter.
- Needle valve function as a flow-controller, and to turn the gas on and off.
- Rotameter consists of a transparent tube and a flow indicator called 'float' or 'bobbin'. This acts as a flow rate monitor.
- Flowmeters are fixed on a florecent background to aid visualization in darkroom.
- The flowmeters are connected to the inlet of 'vaporizer'.

Vaporizers

- Vaporizers are equipments used for delivering vapors of volatile liquid inhalational agents.
- They are agent specific.
- They can either be non calibrated type (concentration delivered to the patient not indicated) e.g. Boyle bottle. Goldman (Fig. 8.5) or they can be calibrated type– where a known concentration can be delivered to the patient e.g. ethertec, fluotec, tritec (Figs 8.6a to f) called 'Tec' type vaporizers.

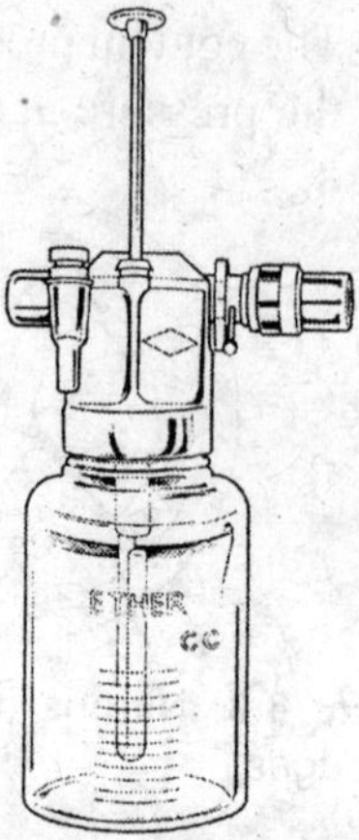

Fig. 8.5: Boyle's bottle

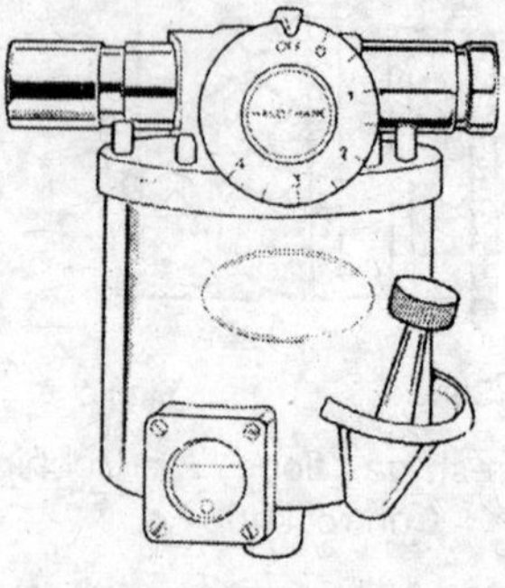

Fig. 8.6a: Fluotec Mk II

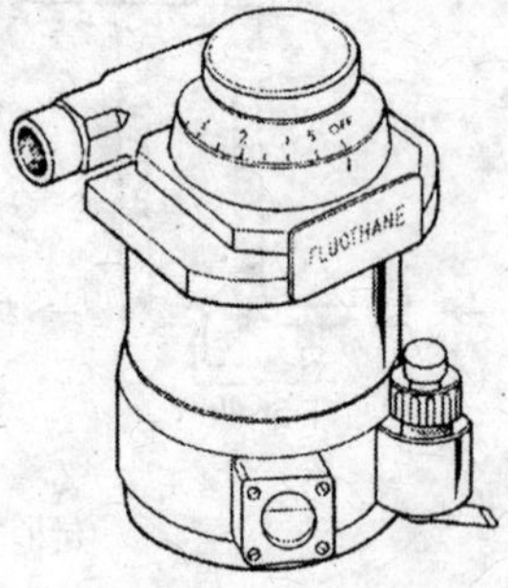

Fig. 8.6b: Fluotec Mk III

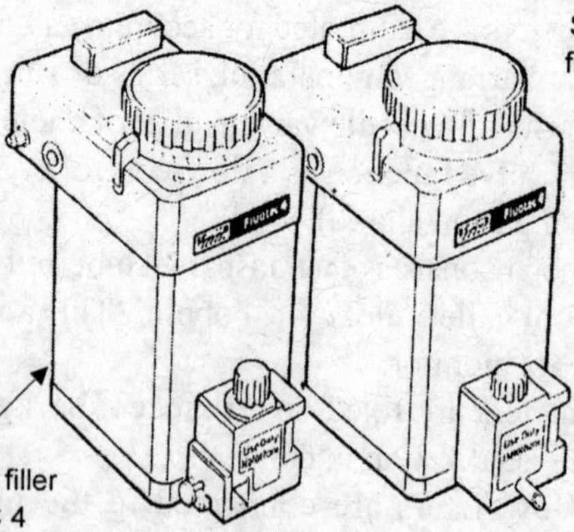

Fig. 8.6c: Keyed filler and screw cap filler

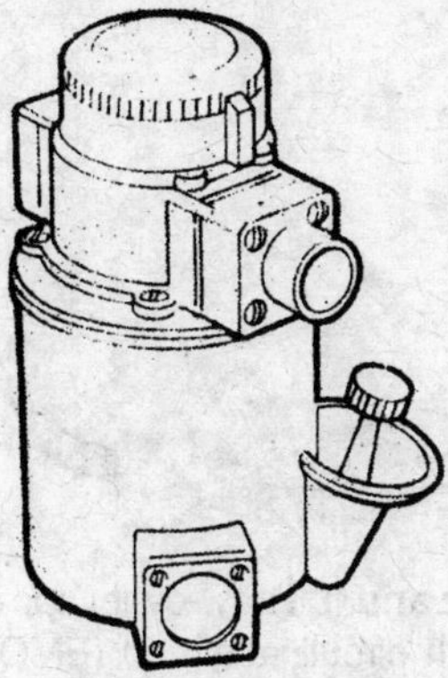

Fig. 8.6d: Screw cap filler for Diethyl-Ether

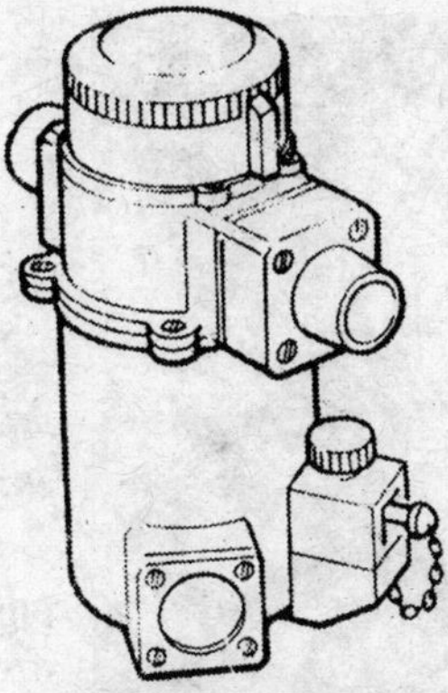

Fig. 8.6e: Keyed filler for Enflurane, Halothane

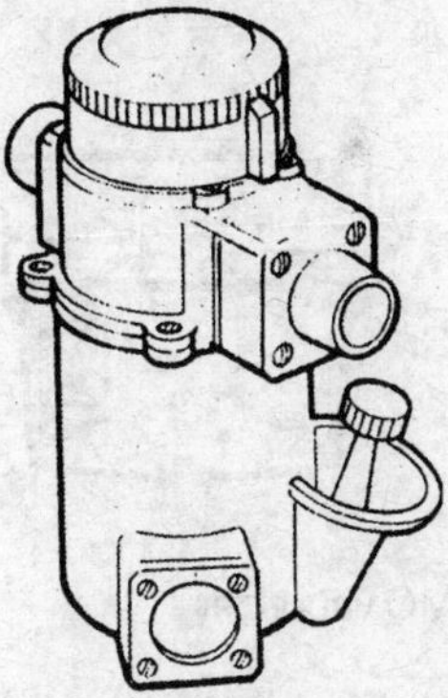

Fig. 8.6f: Screw cap filler for Enflurane, Halothane, Trichoroethylene

- Before filling the anaesthetic agent into the vaporizer, the agent should be confirmed.
- Servicing of the vaporizers should be carried out periodically and the calibration verified.
- Vaporizers like the E.M.O. and OMV air is being drawn over the liquid in the vaporizer, by patient's own respiration or bellows may be used to draw air over the liquid (Figs 8.7 to 8.9d).

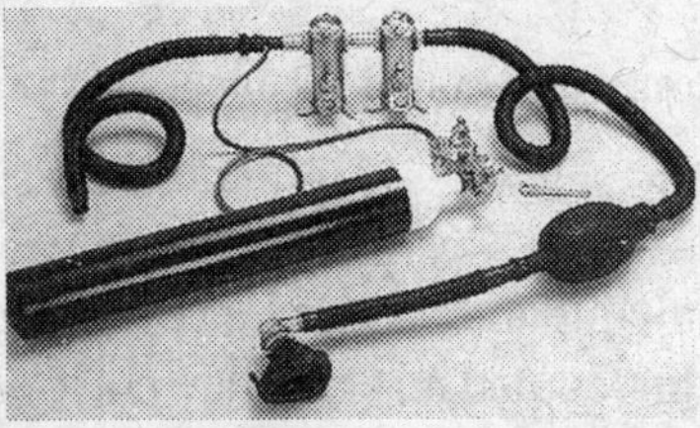

Fig. 8.7: Simple anaesthesia machine

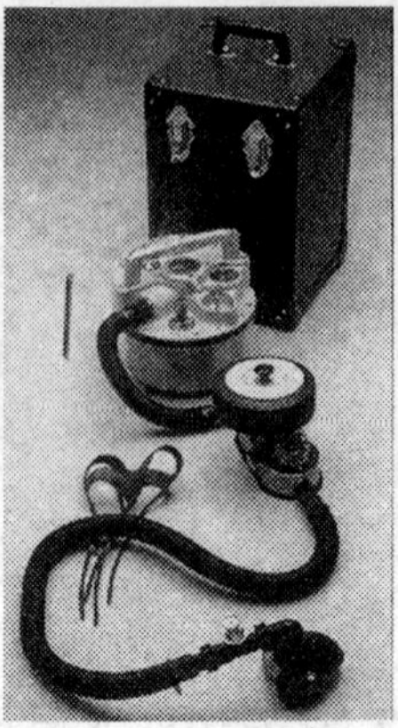

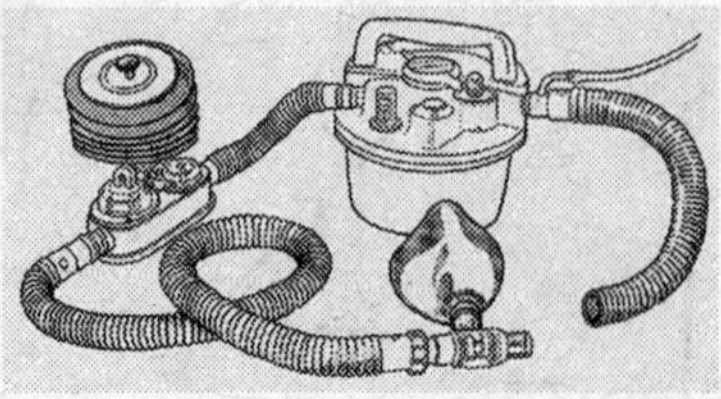

Figs 8.8a and b: Draw-over vaporizer with circuit attached (EMO system)

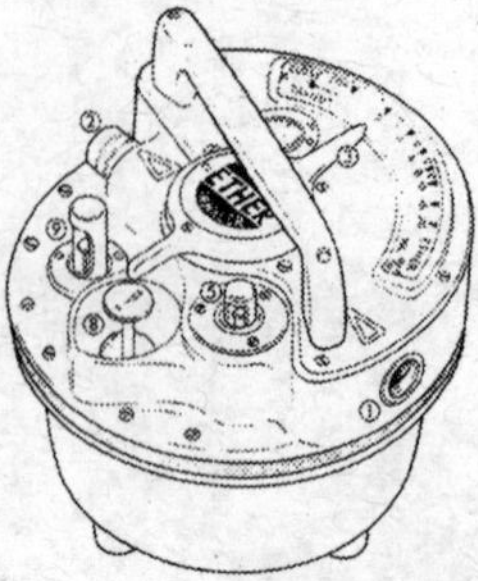

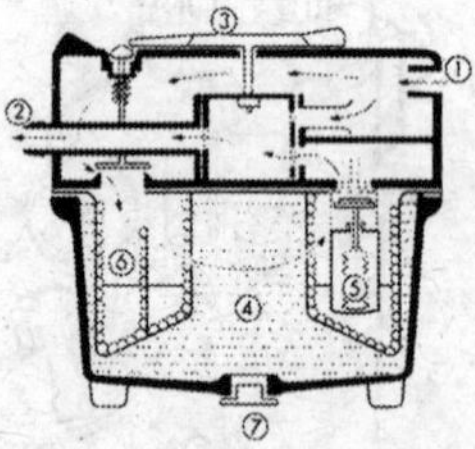

Figs 8.9a and b: EMO vaporizer

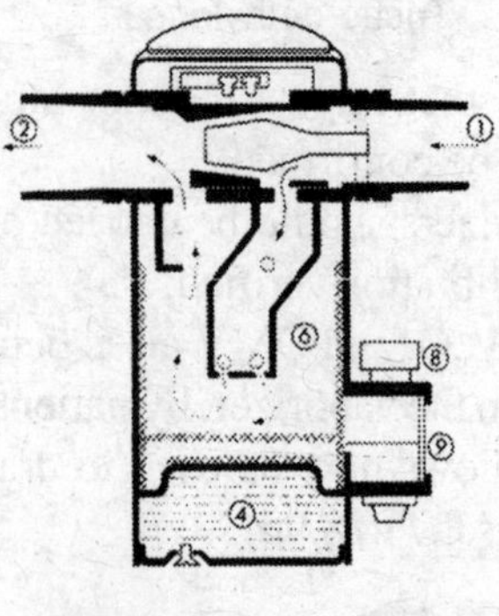

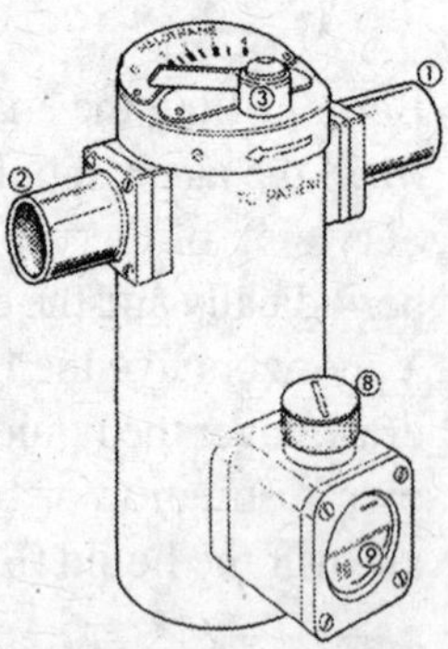

Figs 8.9c and d: Oxford miniature vaporizer (OMV)

- This type of anaesthesia system is very simple and portable.
- This is suitable in abnormal environments where heavy cylinders and machines are not available like at high altitudes.

Breathing Circuits

- The gases and vapors are delivered to the patient through anaesthesia circuits (also called breathing circuits or breathing system).
- This is the system through which oxygenation and carbondioxide removal of the patient is achieved.
- This system consists of (Figs 8.10a to i):
  - Reservoir bag
  - Corrugated tubing from the gas outlet of machine
  - Valves
  - Angle connection
  - Face mask
  - Endotracheal mount and connection
  - Attachment to monitoring equipments from patient and machine.

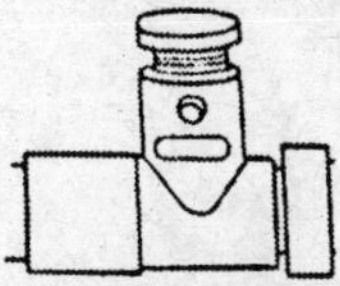

Fig. 8.10a: Spring loaded expiratory valve

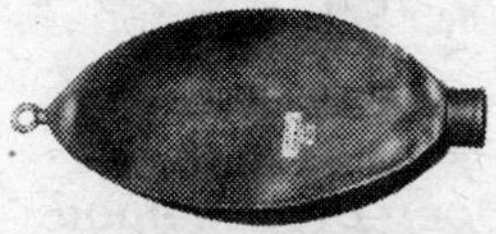

Fig. 8.10b: Rebreathing bag/reservior bag

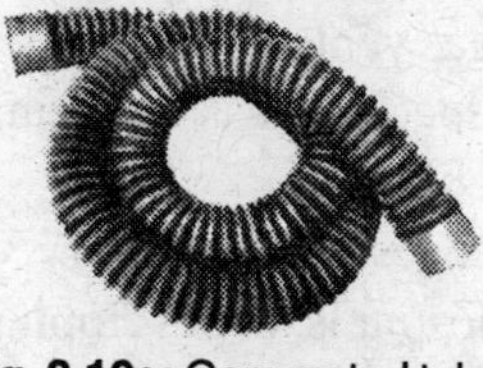

Fig. 8.10c: Corrugated tube

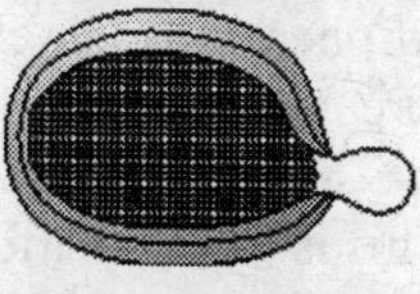

Fig. 8.10d: Schimmel bush mask for open drop method

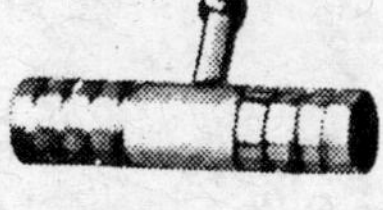

Fig. 8.10e: T-piece

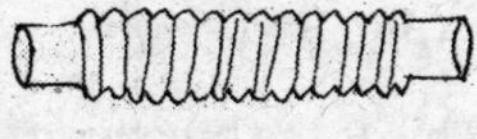

Fig. 8.10f: Flexible calheter mount (Rubber or plastic)

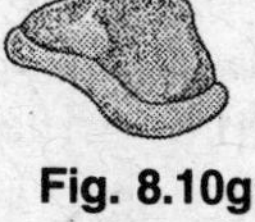

Fig. 8.10g: Angle correction with facemask

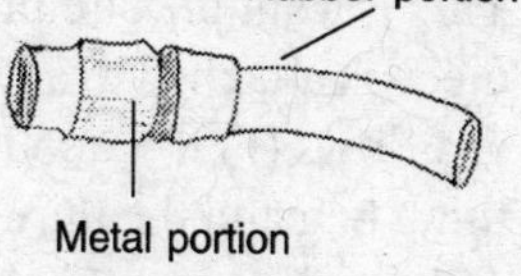

Fig. 8.10h: Calhter mount

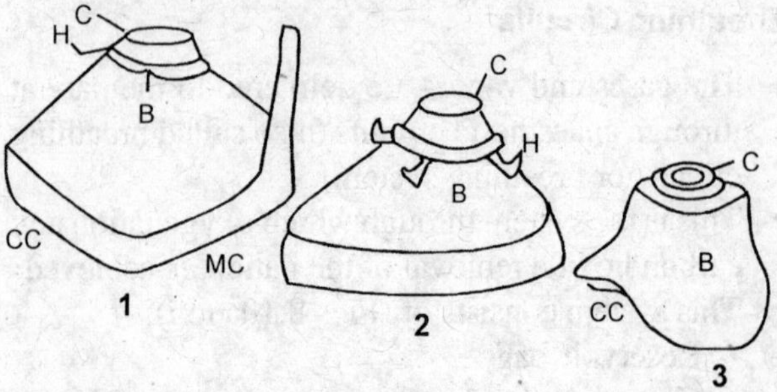

Fig. 8.10i: Face masks—(1) Anatomic rubber mask, (2) Transparent disposable mask and (3) Rendell baker-soucek mask

- Ancillary devices–humidifiers, spirometers, pressure gauges, filters, gas analyzers, sodalime cannister, waste gas scavengers etc.
  - There are different types of breathing circuits.
  - The systems used in different breathing circuits are different.

Anaesthetic Systems

i. Open Drop Method

In the open systems, the patient inhales the anaesthetic agent delivered by open drop and the carrier gas being atmospheric air. The expired gas vented to the atmosphere directly. It requires a special mask covering with 6-8 layers of gauze (Fig. 8.10d).

- This is a simplest form of anaesthesia delivery.
- This is still used in district hospitals, in developing countries, where essential machine is not available.

ii. T–piece System

- This is the breathing circuit used for neonates and children.
- Children weighing up to 20 kg this circuit is used.
- This is a simple circuit in which one limb of a 'T' piece is attached to a light weight tubing for fresh gas flows (FGF), another limb attached to a breathing bag and the third to the patient (Fig. 8.10e).
- This is further modified as shown in (Figs 8.11 and 8.12).

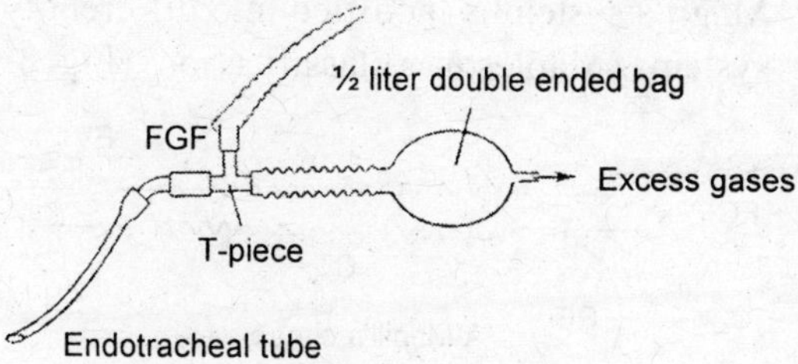

Fig. 8.11: Rees' modification of Ayre's T piece (Mapleson F)

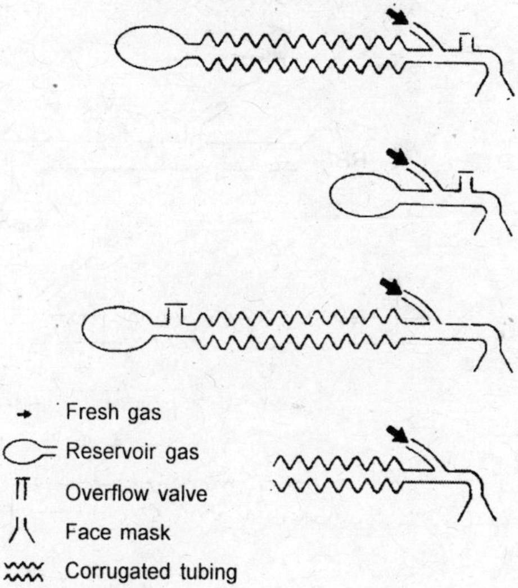

Fig. 8.12: T piece modifications

- 2-2½ times minute volume flows should be used with this system.

iii. Magills system

- Consists of fresh gas flow inlet near the reservoir bag (Fig. 8.1).
- Reservoir bag attached to the corrugated tubing- which is about 1 metre long.
- The other end of the corrugated tubing is attached to a relief valve or expiratory valve.
- Relief valve is attached to either to a face mask with angle connection or to the endotracheal mount connection.

- Magills system is modified into different type of systems (Mapleson's classification) (Fig. 8.13).

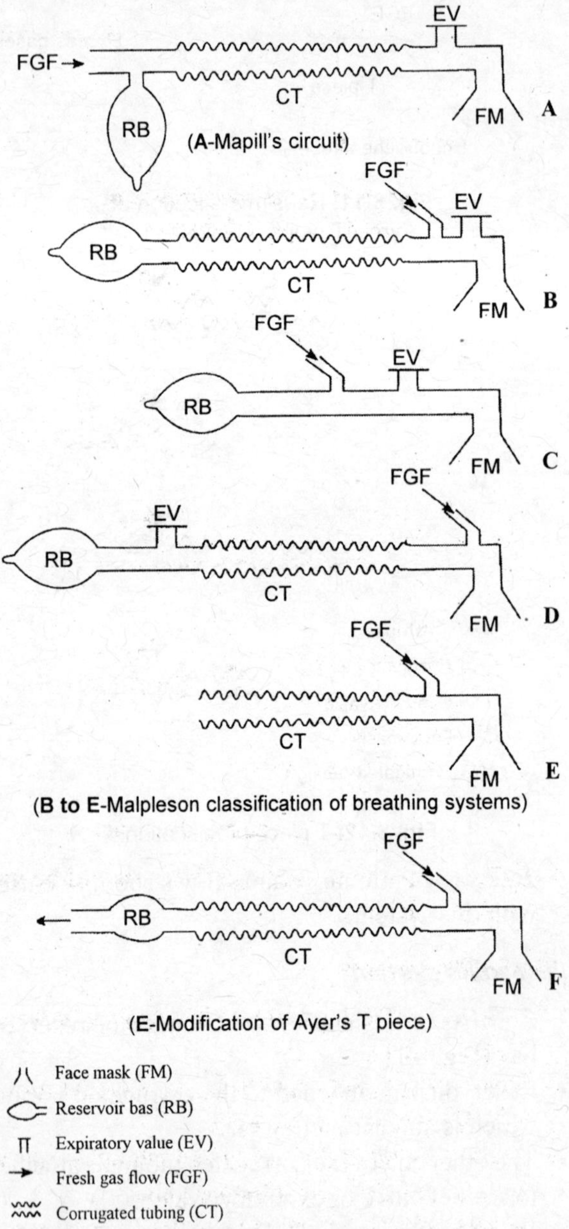

Fig. 8.13: Anaesthesia circuits

- All these systems require high gas flows.
- This circuit is available as non-disposable item made of antistatic black corrugated rubber tubing or disposable, transparent, plastic tubing, for single use.

Bain Co-axial Circuits

- It is one of the modified coaxial system of Mapleson D Circuit (Fig. 8.14).

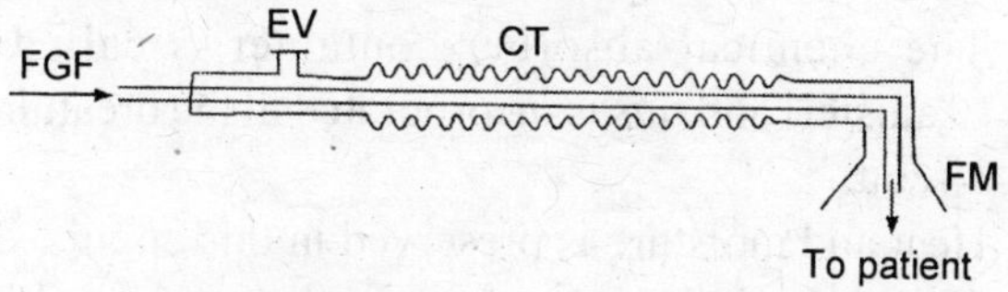

Fig. 8.14: Bain circuit (Coaxial Mapleson D)

- The fresh gases enter the system by means of a narrow–bore inflow tube which lies within a corrugated tubing.
- Patients expired gas–which contain carbondioxide (CO_2) is vented outside the atmosphere partially.
- The corrugated tubing is light weight.
- It can be used in all age groups.
- It is very convenient for all anaesthetic procedures especially for head and neck surgeries.
- High fresh gas flow (70 ml/kg/min) are required both for spontaneous and controlled ventilation.
- This can be used along with several types of anaesthesia ventilators.

Closed System or Circle System

Closed system or circle system with carbondioxide absorption (two phase system):

- An inspiratory and expiratory tubes are used. The exhaled CO_2 is removed by chemical absorption (Sodalime or Baralime).
- Circle system have two unidirectional valves one each on inspiratory and expiratory limb.
- This circuit is attached to the patient by a 'Y'-connector (Fig. 8.15).

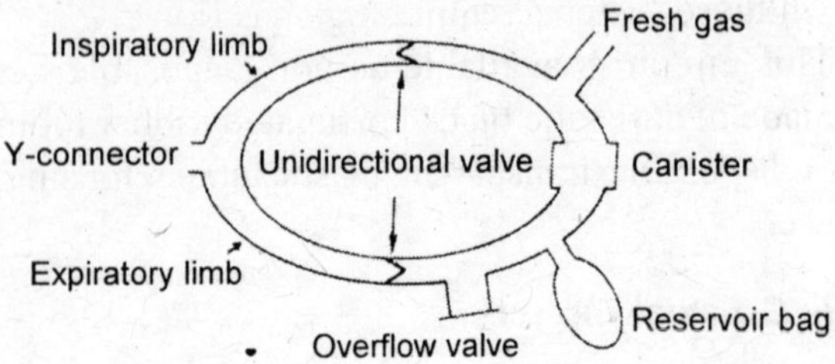

Fig. 8.15: Components of circle system

- The chemical absorber container is called a 'Canister' and this is incorporated in the breathing circuit.
- Heat and moisture is preserved in this circuit.
- This circuit is economical when agents like isoflurane or enflurane is used.
- Low flow can be used with this 'circuit'.

***To and Fro Single Phase System or Circuit:* (Fig. 8.16)**

- Gases pass through the canister during both inspiration and expiration.
- Near the mask (patient), the port for the fresh gas is attached.
- Canister is available in different sizes.
- It is made of metal–so can be sterilized easily.
- Nowadays plastic models are available.
- Since the canister is near to the patient, it is cumersome to use.

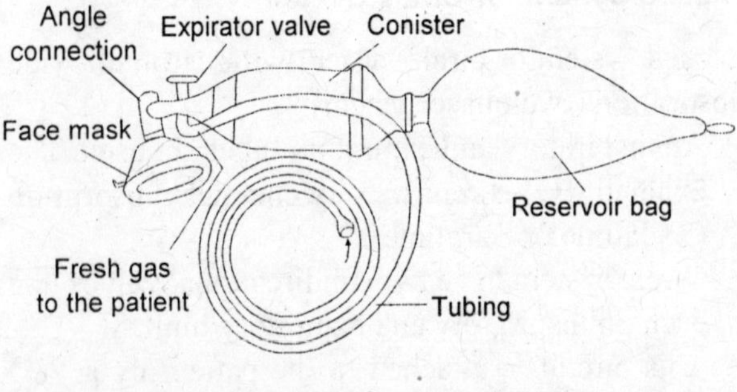

Fig. 8.16: The Water's 'to and fro' sodalime canister

- The chemical used for carbondioxide absorption is either sodalime or baralime.
- Sodalime is a mixture of 90% calcium hydroxide, 5% sodium hydroxide and 1% potassium hydroxide with silica to prevent powdering. Baralime is 80% barium hydroxide.
- Some of the anaesthetic agents are incompatible with sodalime (like trichloroethylene) and should not be used along with sodalime.

Connections to Breathing Circuit and Patient

- The breathing circuit is attached to the patient to a face mask.
- Or to an endotracheal tube.
  - Or to a nasopharyngeal airway.
  - The breathing system attached to a face mask via an 'angle connector' (Figs 8.17 and 8.18).

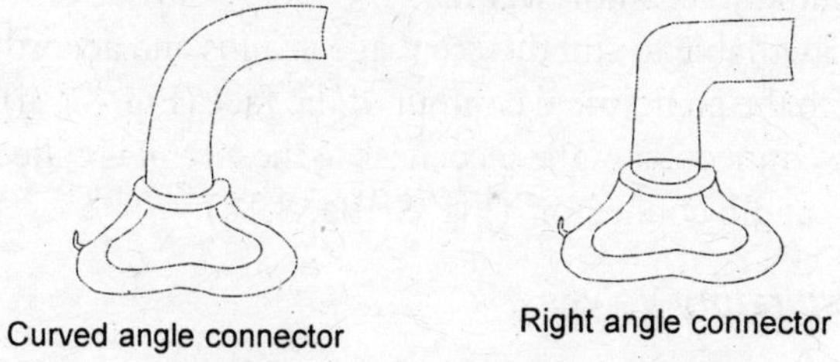

Fig. 8.17: Connector to face mask

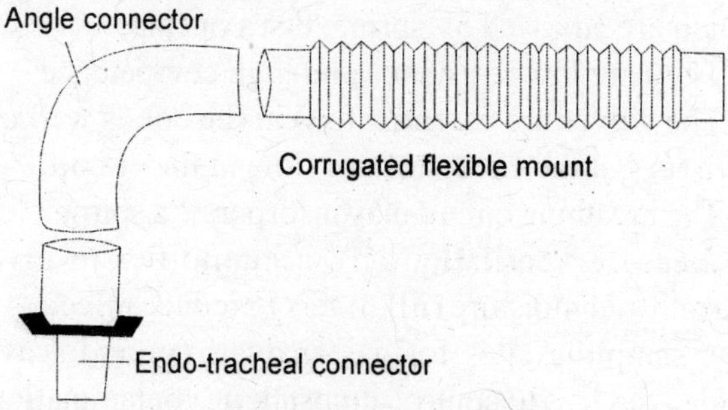

Fig. 8.18: Connectors

- Angle connector can be metal or plastic, right angle or curved type.
- The breathing circuit attached to angle connector is through a 'mount'.

- The mount connection may be plastic or rubber, corrugated or non-corrugated (Figs 8.18, 8.19 and 8.10h).

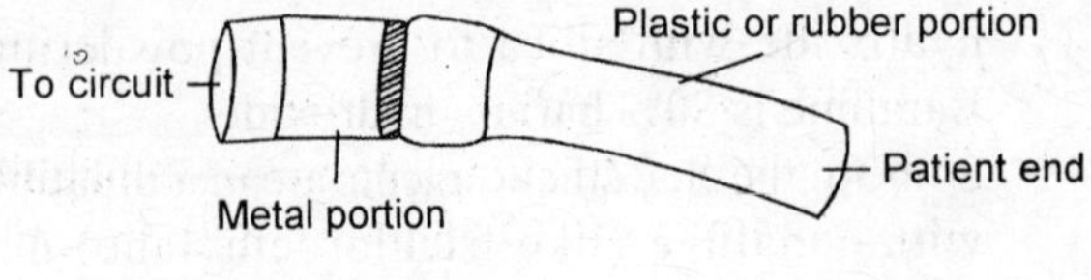

Fig. 8.19: Catheter mount (non corrugated)

- The mount is usually attached with the angle connector, the distal end of which connects to the endotracheal connection.

Face Masks

They are made of rubber or plastic with inflatable or inflated cuff. They are non-disposable items. The pneumatic cushion fits into the face. Various sizes are available to suit different age groups and according to the anatomical contour of the face (Fig. 8.10i). The connection of the face mask to the circuit is called the 'angle connector' (Fig. 8.10g, 8.18).

Respiratory Valves

Unidirectional respiratory valves are incorporated into a breathing circuit in order to direct gas flow which are adjusted by spring, discs or flaps.

- They are low resistance and high competence.
- The valves are essential to vent the co_2 as well as to let out the excess of gas flow in the circuit.

The breathing circuit may incorporate a spirometer to measure ventilation (ii), a humidifier to give warmth and moisture (iii), filters to reduce infections (iv), sampling sites for gas analysis (v) and scavenging devices to control atmospheric contamination by waste gases in the operating room.

9

Tracheal Tubes and Connections

TRACHEAL TUBES

These are both disposable and non-disposable items.

- More commonly are disposable (PVC) which are supplied in sterile packages.
- These are available in different sizes from newborn infant to adult, of internal diameter 2.5 mm to 10 mm.
- Endotracheal tube is attached to a connector at the proximal end which is connected to the breathing circuit.
- The distal end is provided with an inflatable cuff to seal the trachea during controlled ventilation and also to protect the airway from aspiration of stomach or pharyngeal contents.
- Small infants and children the cuff is not provided in tracheal tubes (Fig. 9.1).

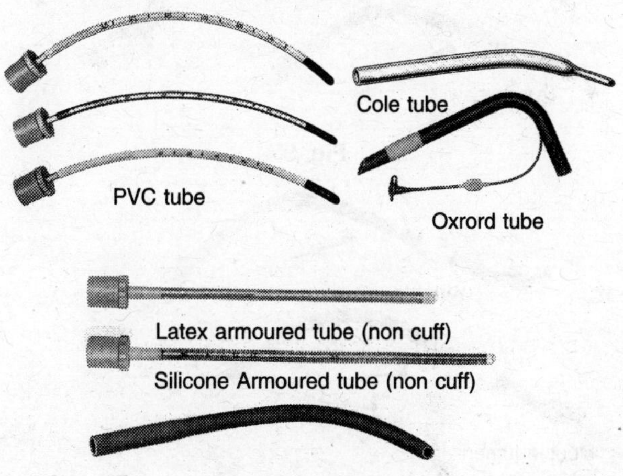

Fig. 9.1: Paediatric tubes

A variety of special tubes are available, namely armoured tubes or reinforced tubes (non-kinkable), double lumen tubes and laser resistant tubes (Figs 9.2 to 9.5). They are all designed for specialised procedures and surgery. Tracheal tubes of different sizes are required. The size quoted usually is the internal diameter (ID).

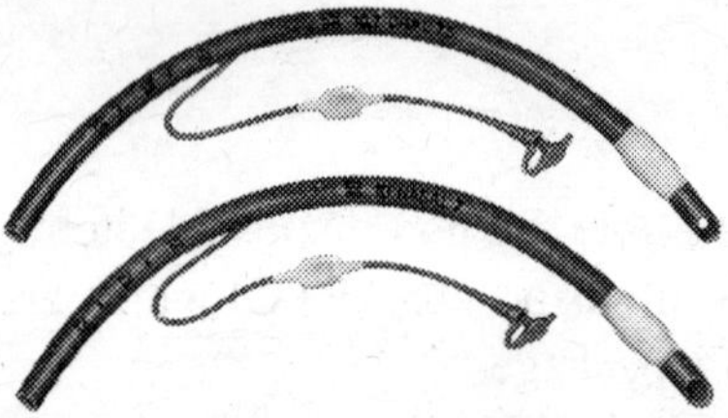

Fig. 9.2: Red rubber cuffed oral and nasal endotracheal tubes

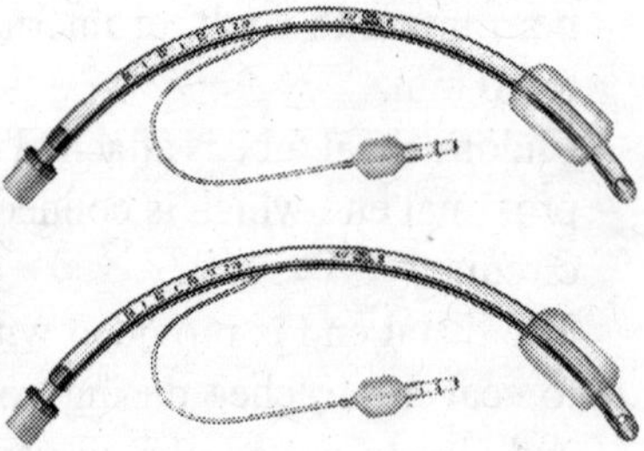

Fig. 9.3: PVC cuffed disposable oral and nasal endotracheal tubes

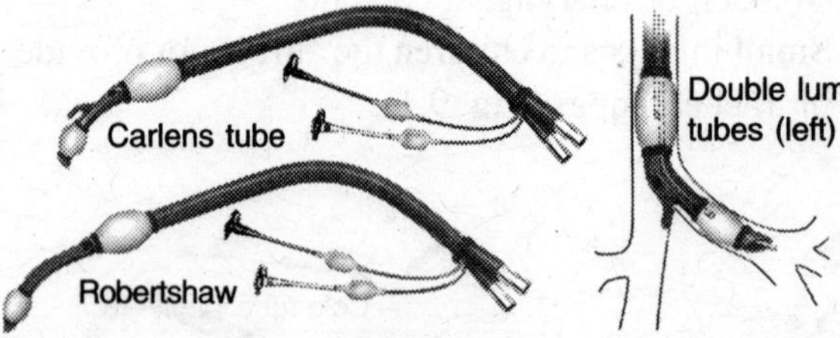

Fig. 9.4

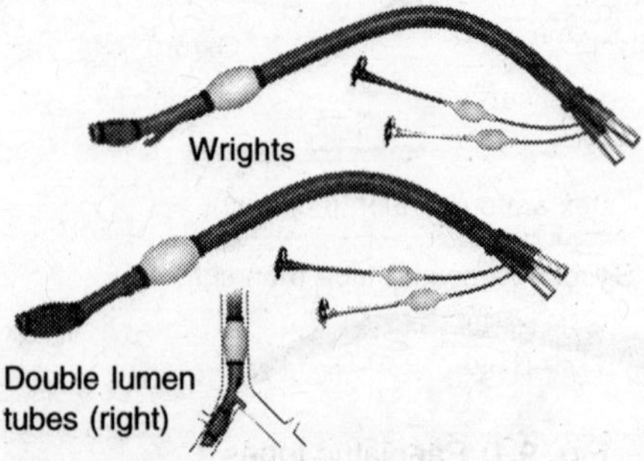

Fig. 9.5

Tube size required in different age is as follows:

Adult Male : 8, 8.5, 9, 9.5, 10 mm ID

Adult Female : 7, 7.5, 8, 8.5 mm ID

Length Oral : 20-23 cm

Paediatric age group size –

$$\frac{\text{Age in years}}{4} + 4 \text{ mm} = \text{ID } (0.5 \pm \text{mm})$$

Paediatric age group length –

$$\frac{\text{Age in years}}{2} + 12 \text{ cm}$$

A tube of one size small ID is required for nasal intubation and the length calculated as:

$$\frac{\text{Age}}{2} + 15 \text{ cm}$$

Suggested Endotracheal Tube Sizes

Age	*Internal Diameter (mm)*
Upto 2 months	2.5 and 3.0
3 to 5 months	3.0 and 3.5
6 to 9 months	3.5 and 4.0
10 months to 1 year	4.0 and 4.5
2 to 4 years	4.5 and 5.0
5 years	5.0 and 5.5
6 to 7 years	5.5 and 6.0
8 to 9 years	6.0 and 6.5
10 years	6.5 and 7.0
11 to 12 years	7.0 and 7.5
13 to 14 years	7.5 and 8.0
> 14 years	7.5, 8.0, 8.5, 9.0

For females 0.5 mm less preferable

Different types of Endotracheal tubes	*Material*
• Plain oral, nasal and cuffed oral and nasal	– Red rubber P.V.C. Latex. Silicone rubber
• Armoured tubes plain and cuffed	– Latex Silicone rubber
• Double lumen tubes (Right side, left side)	– Red rubber or P.V.C.

- Tip configurations of Endotracheal tubes (Fig. 9.6).

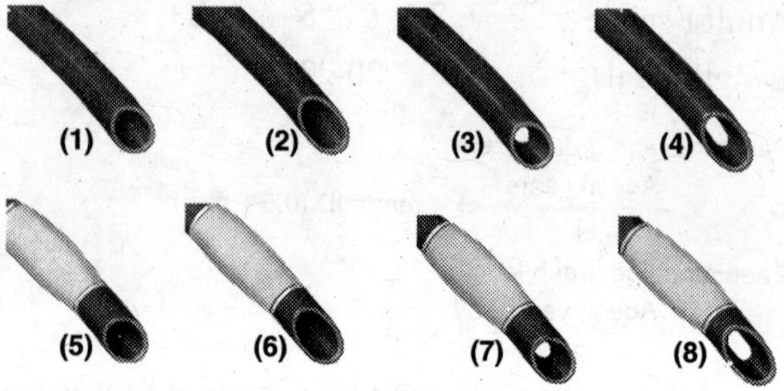

1. Oral without cuff	5. Oral with cuff
2. Nasal without cuff	6. Nasal with cuff
3. Oral with Murphy's eye	7. Oral with cuff with Murphy's eye
4. Nasal with Murphy's eye	8. Nasal with cuff with Murphy's eye

Fig. 9.6: Tip configurations of endotracheal tubes

Different Endotracheal Tubes Characteristics

	Type	*Remarks*
A. Plain oral, nasal Cuffed oral, nasal	Red rubber	* Satisfactory * Relatively inexpensive
	Plastic	* Single use * Expensive
	Latex	* Perish easily * No advantage over red rubber
	Silicone rubber	* Floppy but satisfactory * No advantage over red rubber
B. Armoured tubes	Latex	* Satisfactory * Cheaper than Silicone
	Silicone rubber	* Expensive * Ideal
C. Double Lumen	Red rubber	* Economical * If careful handling can be used several times.
	Plastic	* Disposable * Expensive * Tendency for bronchial cuff to burst.

Endotracheal Tube Connectors

- Tube connectors are different types (Figs 9.7 and 9.8).

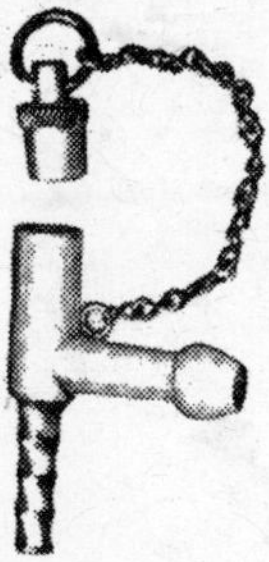

Cob suction union (Metal)

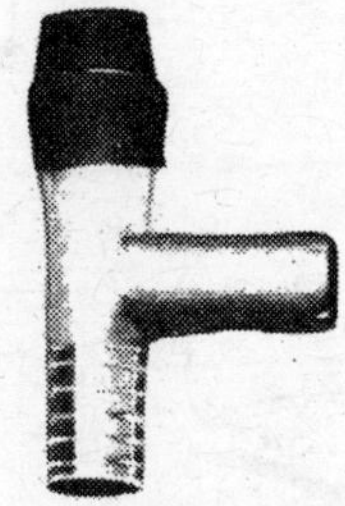

Magill suction union (Metal)

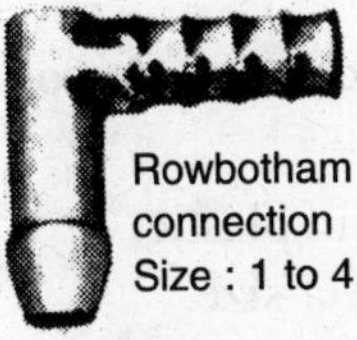

Rowbotham connection Size : 1 to 4 (Metal)

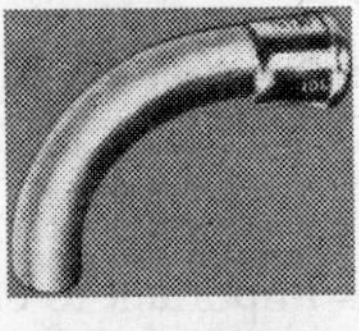

Magill connection (oral)

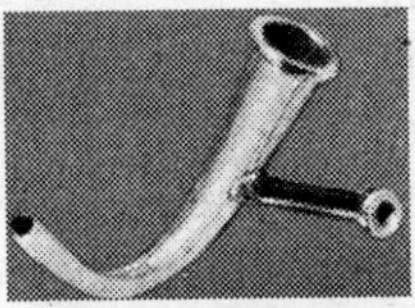

Magill connection nasal

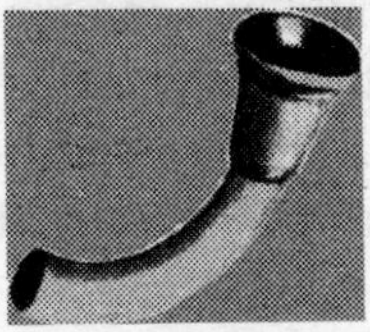

Magill connection nasal

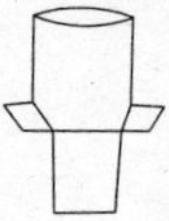

Plastic connector

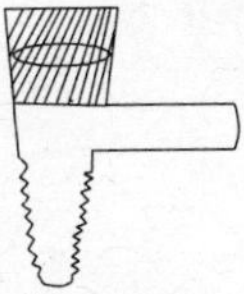

Cob's connector (Metal)

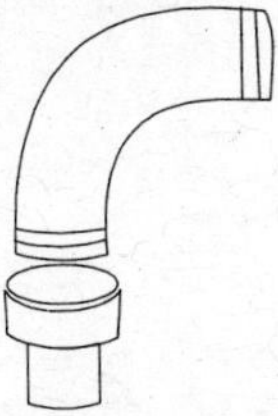

Nose worthy connector (Metal)

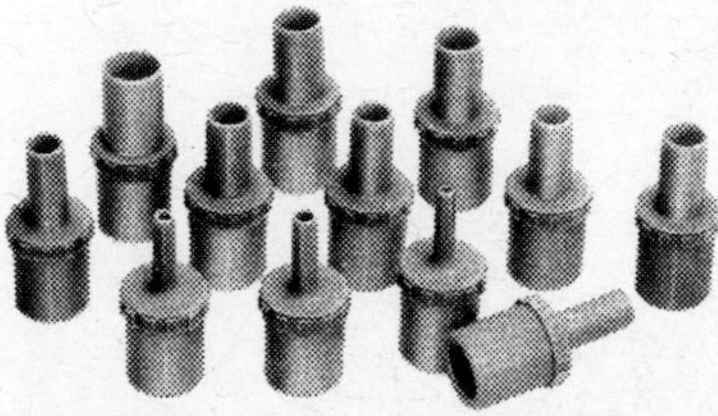

Fig. 9.7: Different endotracheal plastic tube connectors (universal)

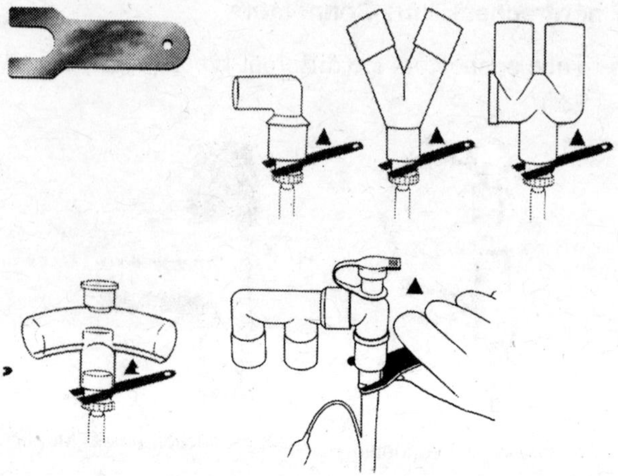

Fig. 9.8: Extraction device for endotracheal connection

- It is available in metal as well as in plastic.
- It is important to choose the correct size.
- The internal diameter of the tube and the connector should be approximately same.
- If the connector is small, there will be increase resistance to the flow of gases.
- In armoured tube, the connector is fitted well into the tube, otherwise the tube may kink at the non spiral proximal portion.

10

Laryngoscopes

It has two major parts—the handle and the blade.

- The handle is a rigid tube containing the battery for the light source.
- There are two basic types of blades–straight and curved. Straight blades are usually used for children and the curved blades are used for adults.

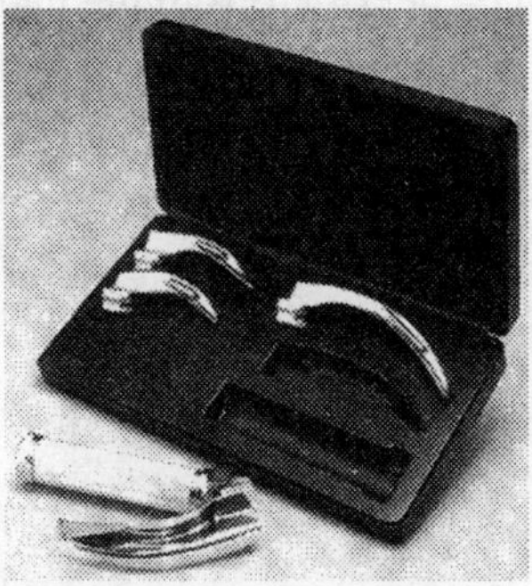

Fig. 10.1: Fibrelight laryngoscopes

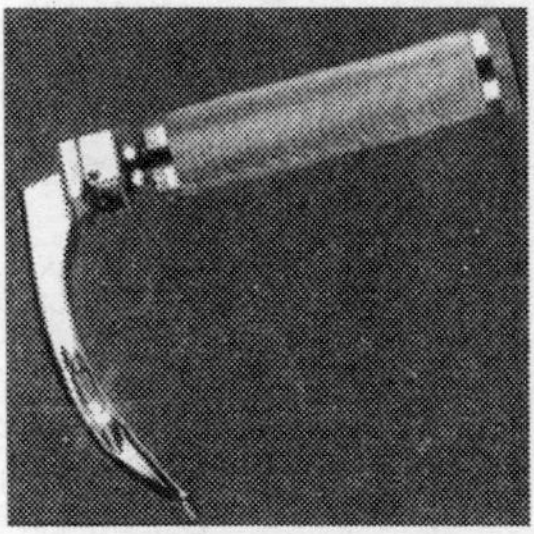

Fig. 10.2: Conventional laryngoscopes

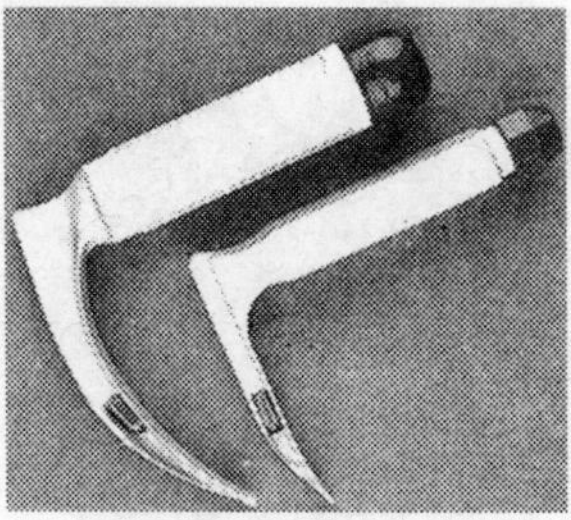

Fig. 10.3: Plastic laryngoscopes

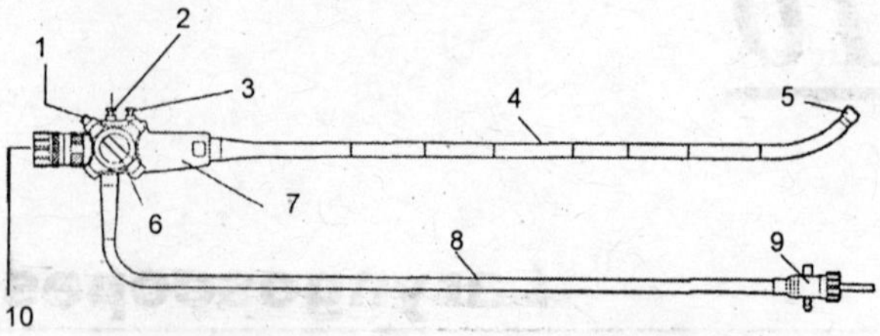

1. Biopsy valve
2. Suction button
3. Air/water button
4. Insertion tube
5. Distal tip
6. Angle control knobs
7. Control body
8. Light guide tube
9. Light guide connector
10. Eyepiece lens

Fig. 10.4: Fibreoptic laryngoscope

- Small, medium, large and extra large blades are available.
- They could be detached from the handle.
- They are interchangeable.
- Flexible fibre optic laryngoscopes are available which is used for difficult intubation (Fig. 10.4).

11

Ventilators and Ventilating Accessories

Ventilators are equipments used to assist or control ventilation. It is useful in operation theatre, wards and intensive care units.

- Mechanical ventilation is achieved by the application of positive pressure to the lungs through a tracheal tube.
- There are variety of ventilators by different manufacturers.
- One should get familiarised with it before use by consulting the 'user handbook' provided by the manufacturer (Fig. 11.1).

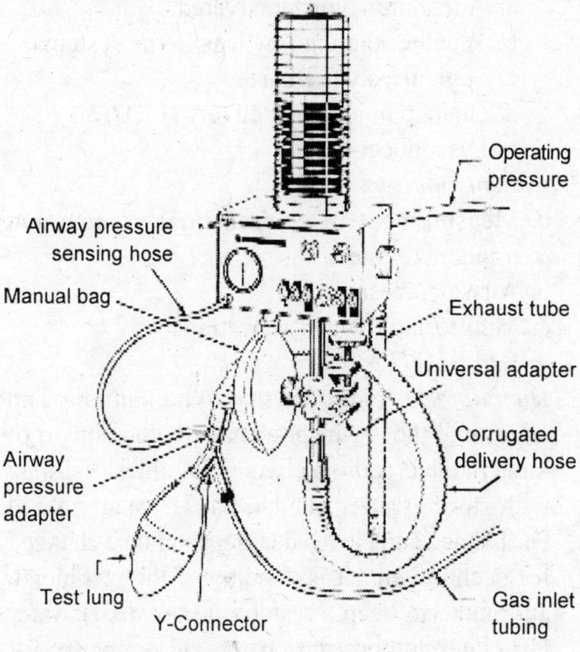

Fig. 11.1: Simple anaesthesia ventilator

A. The ventilators are operated by electricity, battery, compressed gas or manual. The main machine comprises the control knobs for adjusting respiratory rate, inspiratory expiratory ratio, gas flow for tidal and minute ventilation. ICU ventilators have provision for different assist control modes of ventilation like synchronized intermittent mandatory ventilation (SIMV), pressure support ventilation (PSV), addition of continuous positive airway pressures (CPAP) or positive end expiratory pressures (PEEP).

Provision for adjustment of inspired oxygen concentration (FIO_2) is also provided.

VENTILATORY ACCESSORIES

A. *Ventilator monitors:*
  - For adequate ventilation, monitors are incorporated with alarms.
  - This helps to know:
    a. Adequate volume delivered.
    b. Whether there is any leak in the system.
    c. High airway pressure.
    d. Change in oxygen delivery (FIO_2)
    e. Disconnection.

B. *Patient monitors* include:
  a. Measurement of expired tidal volume and minute volume.
  b. Airway pressure.
  c. Monitoring oxygen saturation.
  d. End tidal CO_2.

C. *Humidifiers:* Humidifiers provides humidity and warmth to the dry inspired gas which is incorporated in the breathing circuit. Humidifier is filled with sterile water. The humidifier water should be changed and the inside filter should be changed for each patient. It is the duty of the technician and nurse to keep a watch on humidifier water level intermittently during use. These are used for long term ventilation in ICU and in OT for paediatric patients.

D. *Ventilator tubings:* These are corrugated tubings which are attached to the patient and to the ventilator. There is a tendency to accumulate water inside the tubings during use and intermittently the water collected should be emptied. This item should be cleaned and sterilized after use. It is sterilized after washing in tap water and dipping in 2% glutaraldehyde.

E. *Air Filters:* are used at the ventilator end of breathing system to filter out the atmospheric air. These filters are disposable items.
   - Before use, check the ventilator by attaching to dummy lung or a reservoir bag.
   - Check whether there is any leak or loose connection and the accessory tubings and humidifier is connected properly.

12

Check List for Anaesthesia Machine

All anaesthetic apparatus must be checked before beginning of anaesthesia.

A suitable resuscitation device (for example a self–inflating bag or bellows) to ventilate the lungs of the patient in case the gas supply fails should be available at all times. Operating table should be tiltable.

OXYGEN SUPPLIES

- Cylinder opener (key) should be available at all times.

For Machines Fitted with Cylinder-supply

Turn on the oxygen supply from the cylinder in use and check the pressure (full 2000 1b/sq. inch). Turn on the supply from the reserve cylinder, check the pressure and turn it off again. Check that you have a third cylinder available to replace the cylinder in use when it is exhausted. Keep marker slip on the cylinders as 'Full', 'Empty' or 'In use'.

a. **For machines fitted with a piped gas supply:** Check the source of your piped gas whether it is on. Check that you have a full cylinder of oxygen fitted to your machine in case the piped supply fails.
b. **All machines:** Turn off all gas supplies except one oxygen cylinder or piped supply, open all rotameters. Oxygen should flow through only one rotameter tube (the oxygen only). If this does not happen, do not use the machine.
c. If your machine has an oxygen-failure warning device, test it as follows:

1. Turn on the gas supply from one oxygen cylinder (pipeline disconnected if fitted) and one nitrous oxide cylinder (if fitted).
2. Open rotameter tap to give a flow of oxygen and Nitrous oxide of 5 litres/min.
3. Turn off the oxygen supply at the cylinder. If a functioning warning device is fitted, an alarm should sound as the oxygen failure occurs automatically cuts off the nitrous oxide supply also.
4. After the test remember to open the oxygen cylinder valves again. Open the cylinder valve once and close it before attaching to the machine. This will remove the dust at the valve. Open the valve fully while in use. Never use oil or lubricants on cylinder valve and assembly point.

Avoid using a machine that does not have a functioning oxygen failure alarm. If you have no alternative, you must record the oxygen cylinder pressure every 5 min throughout anaesthesia and change cylinders when the cylinder pressure drops below 1500 kpa (15, atmospheres, 220 p.s.i.) Never begin anaesthesia with a machine that has only a single source of oxygen, i.e. only one cylinder or one pipeline supply.

NITROUS OXIDE

Check the labels. Keep reserve cylinder. The amount present in the cylinder can only be ascertained by weighing as the gas is in liquid form and the gas pressure above the liquid level remains reasonably constant as long as any liquid remains. Till the exhaustion of the cylinder, the pressure will show high, only when all the liquid is vaporized, there will be drop in pressure. Therefore, a cylinder which stores 750 lb/sq. inch, may not be still full. So the cylinder should be labeled ‘Full’, ‘In use’ or ‘Empty’.

ROTAMETERS

Inspect visually for cracks. Make sure that the bobbins do not stick in the tubes.

EMERGENCY OXYGEN

Turn on the emergency oxygen (bypass) button or tap. A high flow of oxygen should be delivered from the gas outlet: Note that this supply does not pass through the oxygen rotameter.

VAPORIZERS

Fill the vaporizer before start of anaesthesia. Empty them by draining at the end of the day.

Check that all vaporizers are firmly connected and filled with the correct anaesthetic agent. Check that all filling ports are firmly closed and that concentration dials are set to zero. A Boyle's bottle should have the lever in off position and the plunger pulled up. See no vapour delivery in 'off' position.

LEAKS

Check your machine for leaks before starting each case or when you suspect. Apply suspect areas with soapy water and watch for bubbles from suspected site. Ensure bobbins are not stuck, and valves mobile.

BREATHING SYSTEM

Check for correct assembly. Make sure that you have:

- Face mask of suitable size.
- Oropharyngeal or nasopharyngeal airway of suitable size and adhesive tapes, and Magill forceps.
- Tested laryngoscope and spare.
- Endotracheal tube of suitable size (test cuff by inflating)
- Tested suction apparatus and suction catheters.
- Table or trolley that can be tilted head-down
- All drugs you may need. Check sodalime.
- All electrical points to ventilators, monitors ana suction apparatus to be checked for any loose contact, disconnection, earthing, open wire.

Pre-operative Check

1. Patient identification and consent check for operation and anaesthesia, side/site of surgery, dentures if any, availability of blood.
2. Availability and functioning of anaesthesia machine, intubation sets, drugs and monitors.
3. Confirmation of operation decided upon for that particular patient.
4. Working suction machine and suction catheters.

STANDARD MONITORING EQUIPMENTS

- Check its electrical connections, proper earthing, cables, calibrations, alarm setting.
- Requirement of any extra specialised monitoring.

Warming Blankets, Fluid Warmers

- For major operations warning blankets and fluid warmer to be kept ready.
- Anaesthesia chart to be kept near the anaesthesia trolley for record keeping.
- Blood requisition forms, emergency drugs, colloid and crystalloid solutions, intravenous canula, threeways, extension tubings should be in adequte supply.
- Check defibrillator everyday.
- Blood specimen bottles, blood requisition and investigation forms for special tests perioperatively required to be kept ready.
- Make available, bolsters, sand bags, props, head-support rings, straps, eye pads, harness, nasogastric tubes, temperature monitor, pressor-infusor, assorted sterile syringes and needles and tray, and IV cannula, syringe labels, assorted life-saving drugs, throat pack, styllete, lignocaine spray, jelly file, scissors, stethoscope, venous tourniquet, arm-supports, sphygmomanometer and right size cuff, breathing bag of right size, regional anaesthesia tray.

13

Induction of Anaesthesia

Objective

- To produce sleep.
- Achieved with inhalation of gases and volatile agents.
- Position–supine

A. INHALATIONAL INDUCTION

Inhalational induction preferred:
- For young children.
- Upper and lower airway obstruction
- Bronchopleural fistula, or empyema, when no accessible veins and due to non–availability of appropriate intravenous induction agents.
- The proposed procedure is explained to the patient before starting.
- Patient connected to ECG, SPO_2, NIBP monitor.
- Intravenous line is always secured before start. Check whether patient can open the mouth and extend, turn, flex the neck.
- Anaesthetic agent chosen along with oxygen is delivered gradually to the face via face mask (Fig. 13.1).

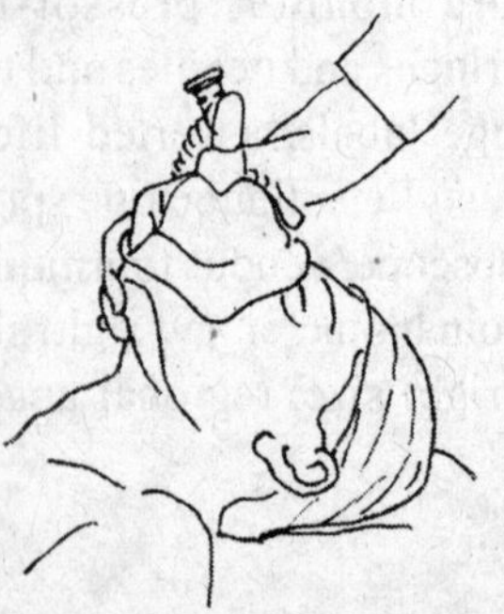

Fig. 13.1: Application of face mask

- In case of children who are not co-operative, the hands and legs are held by one assistant, but not more (that can scare the child).
- Initially, Nitrous Oxide (N_2O) 70% in oxygen is used and flows of gases according to the circuit used.
- Anaesthesia is deepened by the gradual induction of increments of a volatile agent. Halothane 1 to 3 %, Enflurane 1 to 3%, Isoflurane 1 to 3%, one at a time.
- Once the patient is adequately deepened, maintenance levels of halothane 1 to 2%, enflurane 1.5 to 2.5 %, isoflurane 1 to 2% is restored promptly avoid over dosage.
- The induction can be achieved in 20 to 30 seconds.
- Respiration, colour, blood pressure, heart rate monitored during induction.
- Face mask is applied more firmly to avoid leak once the consciousness is lost.
- The airway kept clear manually or when anesthesia is deep enough, by inserting an oral airway.
- If intubation is planned, after attaining adequate depth of anesthesia (relaxed jaw muscles, abdominal muscles) endotracheal tube is secured by direct laryngoscopy.

Preparation

1. Check Anaesthesia machine
2. Check breathing circuits
3. Vaporizer filled for inhalational agent and face masks
4. Keep endotracheal intubation set
5. Keep nasopharyngeal and oropharyngeal airway
6. Keep suction apparatus and catheter
7. Check emergency drug tray
8. IV infusion, canula, spirit and iodine swab, adhesive plaster ready for venepuncture
9. Keep hypodermic needles, syringes, N/G tube

10. Keep patient monitors ready–ECG, SPO_2, $ETCO_2$ and NIBP
11. Check anaesthesia machine monitors.

B. INTRAVENOUS INDUCTION

Objective

- To induce sleep rapidly in the start of anaesthesia.
- Induction is achieved with intravenous agents. (Thiopentone 3-5 mg/kg, Methohexitone 1-1.5 mg/kg, Etomidate 0.3 mg/kg, Propofol 1.5-2.5 mg/kg and Ketamine 2 mg/kg).

Position–Supine

Procedures

Intravenous canula inserted into a peripheral vein, preferably on the dorsum of the left hand and transfusion fluid attached.

- Drugs prepared and labelled (IV agent, muscle relaxant, Atropine).
- Patient connected to the monitor for ECG, non invasive blood pressure (NIBP) and oxygen saturation.
- 100% Oxygen by mask before the drugs are injected.
- Small test dose of intravenous induction agent given and effects observed for any anaphylactic reaction.
- Slow injection of the drug into the vein till the eye lash reflex is obtunded.
- Rapid sequence induction technique used in emergency situation where the stomach is full or chances of regurgitation are a potential problem.
- Anaesthesia maintained with inhalational agent and tracheal intubation done using muscle relaxant.

Preparation

1. Check anaesthesia machine.
2. Check breathing circuits, face mask, intubation set.

3. Keep IV cannula, infusion, spirit and iodine swab, adhesive plaster.
4. Keep drug tray and labels duly fixed on syringes.
5. Keep normal saline bottle for dilution of drugs.
6. Keep induction agents—Thiopentone, Propofol, Ketamine.
7. Keep arm boards, and suction ready.
8. Keep monitors for ECG, SPO_2, NIBP, $ETCO_2$
9. Check anaesthesia machine monitors. Watch colour, pulse, breaths.

14

Tracheal Intubation

Objectives

1. To secure clear airway for anaesthetised patients,
2. In difficult patients like obese, thick jaw, edentulous,
3. Abnormal anatomical airway,
4. Sharing of the airway by surgeons,
5. Protection of airway from regurgitaion of stomach contents and aspiration,
6. To aid in assist and control of ventilation when muscle relaxants are used,
7. To facilitate suction of respiratory tract,
8. To prevent collapse of lungs in thoracic operations, and
9. For prolonged anaesthesia.

LARYNGOSCOPY AND INTUBATION

Position for Laryngoscopy and Intubation

Flexion of the head at the neck and extension of the head at the atlanto occupital level, the so called 'sniffing' position (Figs 14.1a, 14.1b and 14.2).

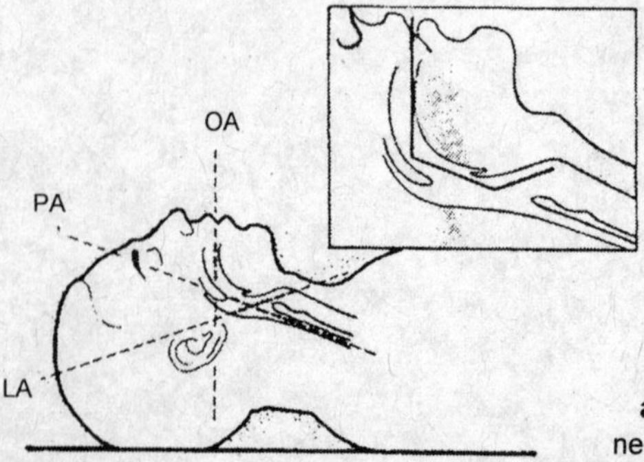

a. Head on neutral position

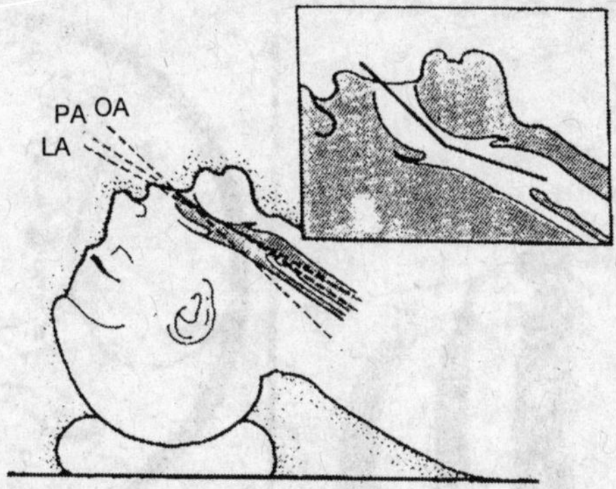

b. Head elevated on pad, head extended on neck (sniff position)

OA = Oral axis
PA = Pharyngeal axis
LA = Laryngeal axis

Figs 14.1a and b: Head position and the Axes of the upper airway

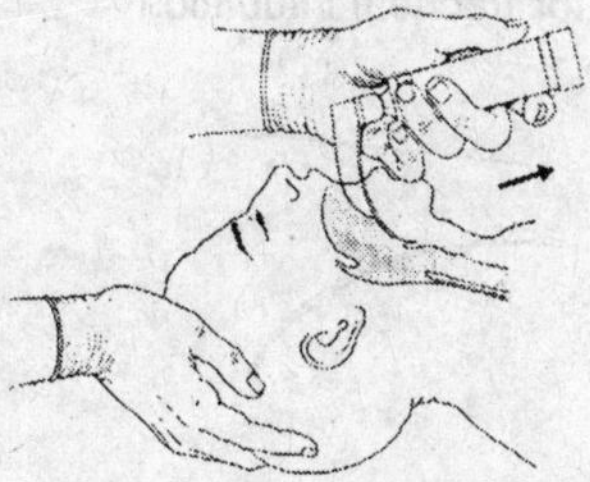

Fig. 14.2: Direct laryngoscopy

- The head is elevated placing a low pillow or ring. Oral cavity axis (OS), pharyngeal, axis (PA) and laryngeal axis (LA) are different. In this all three axes bring into alignment position and vocal cords will be viewed best with laryngoscopy.

Things required for laryngoscopy and intubation (Fig. 14.3):

- Laryngoscope battery handle.
- Curved and staight blade (all sizes) and extra large blade.
- Endotracheal tubes
- 5 ml syringe
- Malleable stylet and Magill's forceps (Fig. 14.4)
- Oropharynged/Nasopharynged airway

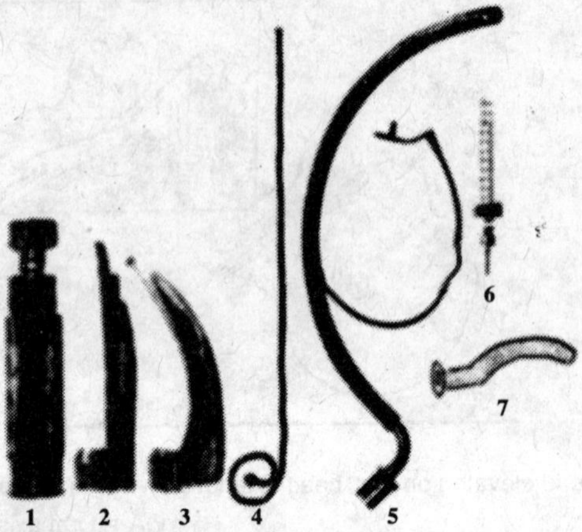

1. Laryngoscope battery handle
2. Straight blade
3. Curved blade
4. Malleable stylet
5. Endotracheal tube
6. Syringe to inflate tube cuff
7. Oropharyngeal airway

Fig. 14.3: Equipment for tracheal intubation

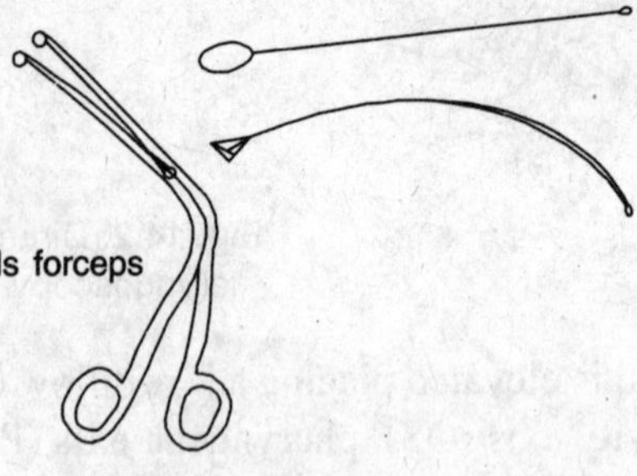

Fig. 14.4: Malleable endotracheal stylets and Magill's forceps

- If difficult intubation is anticipated following additional things to be kept ready:
  - MacCoy Laryngoscope
  - LMA
  - 6 mm intubating bougie
  - Fibreoptic laryngoscope
  - Xylocaine jelly, sterile gauze pieces
- Intubation can be by orally or nasally

- It can be direct visualing larynx by using laryngoscope and intubation or
- Blind intubation where the mouth opening is restricted or laryngoscope not available
- Difficult intubation is done with the help of fibreoptic laryngoscope.

THROAT PACKING

It is done to prevent secretion and blood entering into the respiratory tract during nasal and oral surgeries, and prevent air leak.

- The pack is done after the endotracheal tube is secured in position.
- It is done with a sterile, soft, absorbent, specially made ribbon gauze 1-1.5 cm width.
- Under direct vision using laryngoscope with the help of Magill's forceps pack is inserted.
- It is done around the tube.
- It should not be too loose or too tight.
- The pack to be removed, once the operation/procedure is over.

15

Airway Management with Face Masks

- Maintenance of airway is important in an unconscious patient.
- It is achieved by tilting the head backwards, displacing the mandible forward and opening the mouth (Fig.15.1).

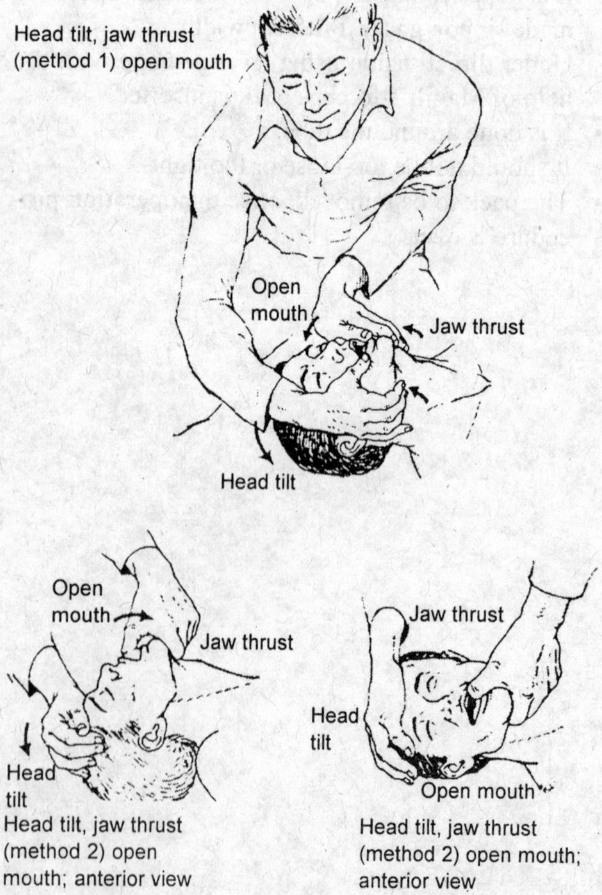

Fig. 15.1

- For inhalation anaesthesia, oxygen administration and for assisting respiration the airway should be clear.
- During CPR, bag and face mask ventilation can be provided through AMBU bag (artificial mechanical breathing unit)–or by using anaesthesia machine.
- The face mask should form a tight seal on the patient's face while fitting comfortably in the users hand.
- The thumb and index finger of the left hand on the body of the mask to push the mask downward on the face. The remaining fingers placed on the mandible.
- While applying the mask on the face, the eyes to be protected.
- Select the appropriate size and shape for different facial characteristics (e.g., fat, emaciated, Oedentulous, prominent nares, burns, flat nose, receding jaws, beard, nasogastric tube, nasal pack etc.).
- To maintain airway, use of nasal or oral airways may be required.

16

Laryngeal Mask Airway (LMA) and Other Airways

LARYNGEAL MASK AIRWAY (LMA)

- LMA is a non-invasive airway.
- It is made of medical grade silicone rubber.
- It is reusable after sterilization by steam autoclaving.
- It has a mask at the distal end with inflatable outer rim.
- The mask sits in the hypopharynx, just above the larynx.
- The mask is extended to a tube, which is attached to the breathing circuit.
- Different types and sizes of LMA are available (LMA–classic, flexible, fastrach, unique etc.) (Fig. 16.1).

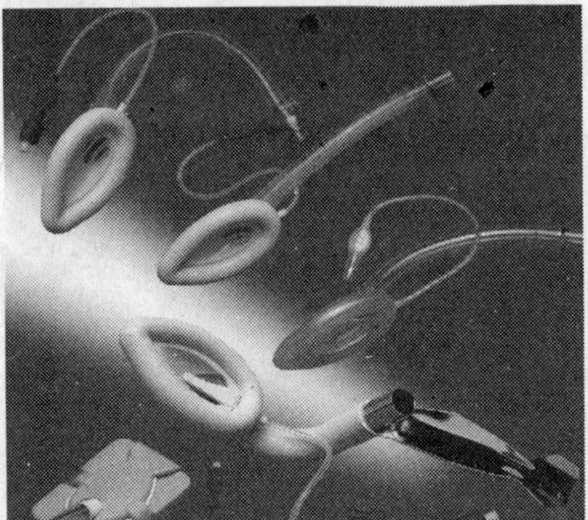

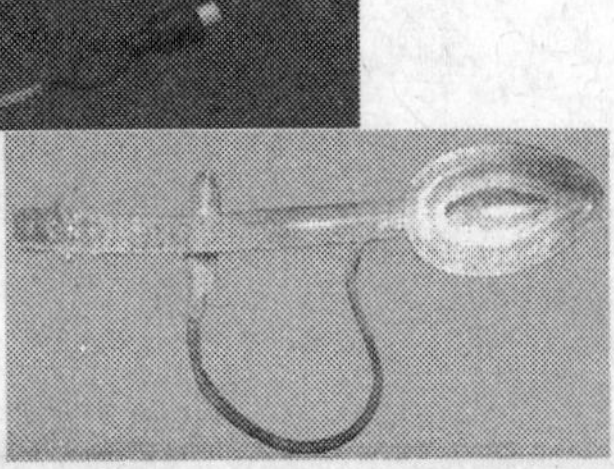

Fig. 16.1: Laryngeal mask airways

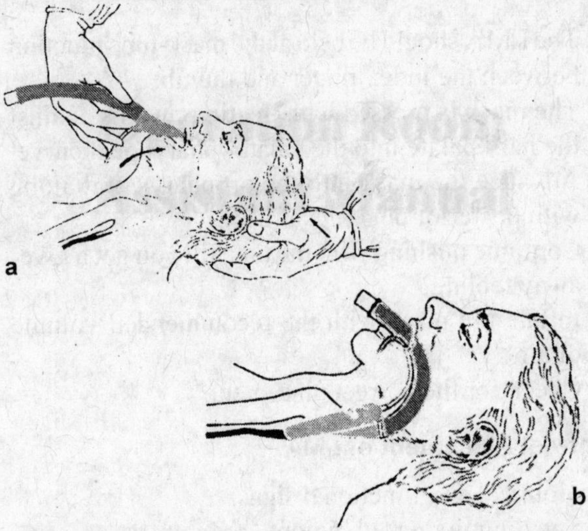

Fig. 16.2: a. LMA-insertion and **b.** LMA-in position

- LMA insertion is carried out with the head in the sniffing position, with slight additional head extension or with head in neutral position (Fig. 16.2).
- Seven sizes of LMA-classic and five sizes of flexible are available (Table 16.1).

Table 16.1: LMA sizes—seven sizes of *LMA-Classic* and five sizes of *LMA-Flexible* are available

LMA-Classic		**LMA-Flexible**	
Size	*Patient*	*Size*	*Patient*
1	Neonates/infants upto 5 kg	2	Infants/children 10-20 kg
1½	Intants 5-10 kg	2½	Children 20-30 kg
2	Infants/children 10-20 kg	3	Children over 30 kg/small adults
2½	Children 20-30 kg	4	Normal adults
3	Children over 30 kg/small adults	5	Large adults
4	Normal adults		
5	Large adults		

- Appropriate LMA size to be chosen.
- It should be inserted under general anaesthesia or topical anaesthesia.
- The cuff of the mask should be fully deflated and lubricated at the posterior aspect.

- The LMA should be held at the mask-tube junction between the index finger and thumb.
- The mask is pressed with the tip upwards against the hard palate into the palato- pharyngeal curve.
- Advance the mask into the oropharyx and along with posterior pharyngeal wall.
- Continue pushing with the tube till you get a give-away feeling.
- Inflate the mask with the recommended volume of air.
- Check for the correct placement.

Correct Placement of LMA

Anatomical and functional signs:

- Swelling in thyroid region.
- Outward movement of LMA tube at inflation.
- Cuff of LMA not visible at mouth.
- Tube protruding < 8 cm above teeth.
- Black marking at midline.
- Permits ventilation without any obstruction.
- Positive Capnographic reading.
- Breath sounds on auscultation.

Fixation and Stabilization OF LMA

- Before fixing, insert an appropriate bite block.
- Use adhesive tapes.
- Fix one end to the maxilla, take a round on the LMA and fix to the opposite maxilla.
- Can be fixed to the lower chin also.
- The LMA are re-usable devices which can be cleaned and steam sterilised several times.

Other Airways

- Airways are accessories or adjuncts to maintain a patent respiratory passage and facilitate ventilation.
- It can be supraglottic or infraglottic.
- Supraglottic adjuncts are placed above the glottis e.g.: Oropharyngeal airway (Guedel airway), nasopharyngeal airway, cuffed oropharyngeal airway, laryngeal mask airway, Safars airway, Brook's airway etc.

- Infraglothic airways are the ones which are placed below the level of glottis e.g. Endotracheal tube, combitube, oesophageal airway, tracheostony, tube etc.
- Several modifications of the airways are available to facilitate ventilation and oxygenation.
- Oropharyngeal airway (reusable and disposable). Available in red rubber, plastic or silicone. It has a flange, bite portion and a curved air channel. It is placed orally (Fig. 16.3).

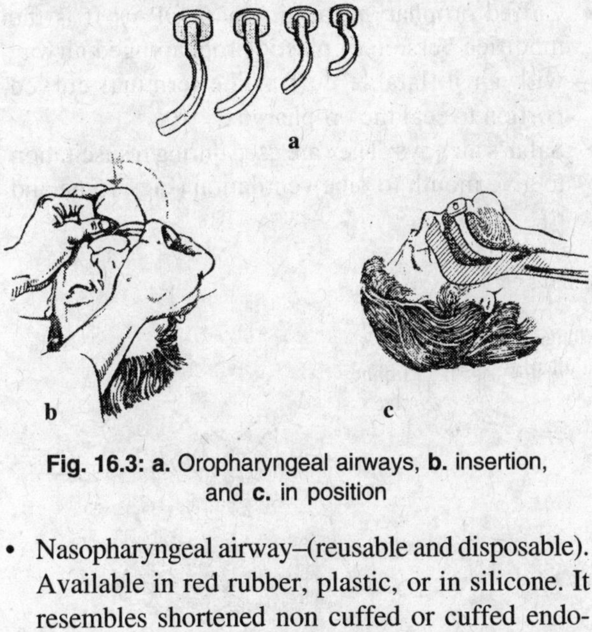

Fig. 16.3: **a.** Oropharyngeal airways, **b.** insertion, and **c.** in position

- Nasopharyngeal airway–(reusable and disposable). Available in red rubber, plastic, or in silicone. It resembles shortened non cuffed or cuffed endotracheal tube, with small flange without a bite portion. It is placed nasally. Binasal combined airways are also available (Figs 16.4 and 16.5).

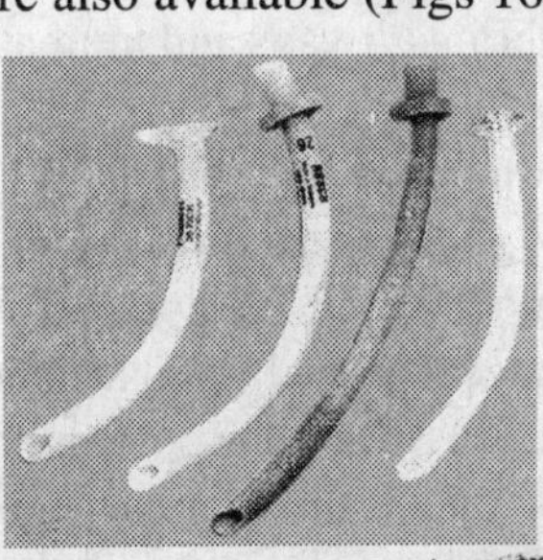

Fig. 16.4: Nasopharyngeal airways

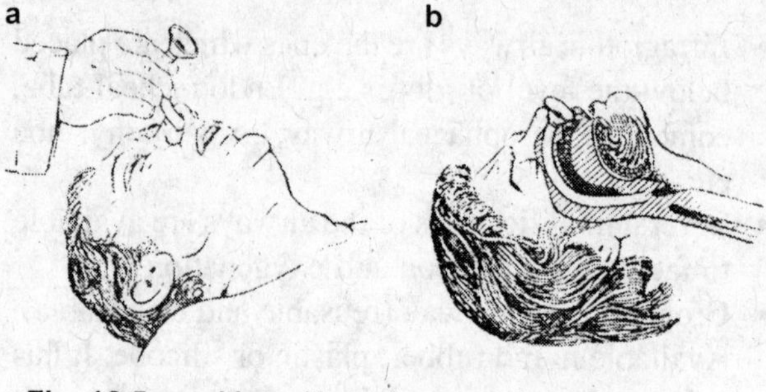

Fig. 16.5a and b: a. Nasopharyngeal airway insertion and **b.** in position

- Cuffed oropharyngeal airway (COPA): It is the modified version of plastic oropharynged airway with an inflatable cuff at the terminal curved portion to seal the oropharynx.
- Safar's airways: They are used during resuscitation to give mouth to tube ventilation (Figs 16.6a and b).

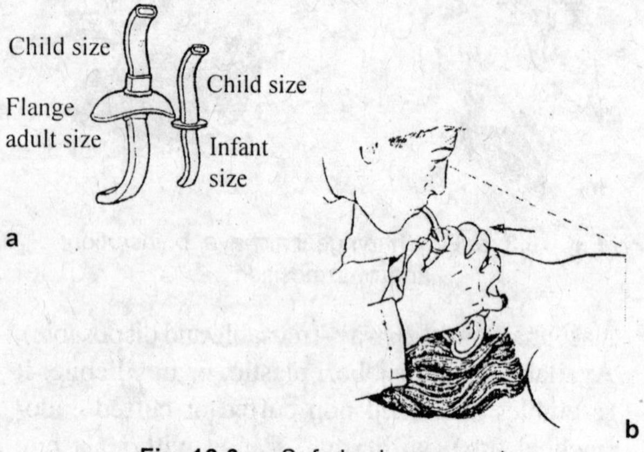

Fig. 16.6: a. Safar's airways, and **b.** in position and in use

- Tongue retracting airways and intubating airways are also available.
- Combitube: It is used during CPR. It does not require laryngoscope for insertion. It has two separate lumen which allows ventilation with either oesophageal or tracheal placement. One tube is occluded at the tip and the other is patent. There are two cuffs, one at the oropharyngeal position, one at the distal end. In-between the two cuffs,

holes are present which are above the glottis to force air or oxygen into the larynx if the tube is placed in the oesophagns (Figs 16.7a to c).

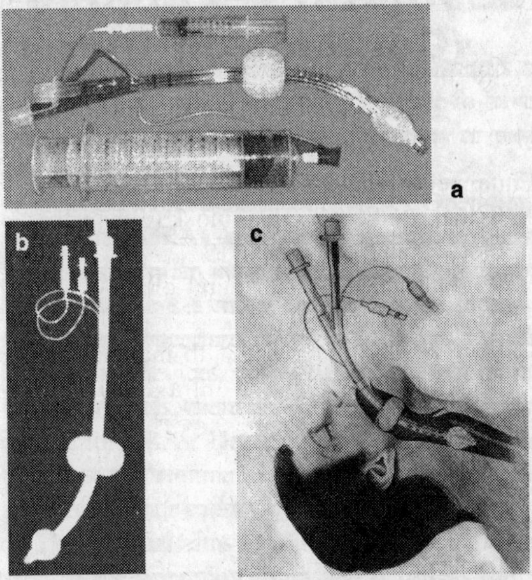

Figs 16.7a to c: Combitubes—**a.** with inflated cuff with syringe, **b.** tracheal and oesophageal tube, and **c.** is placed in the oesophagus

- Oesophageal obturator is placed in the oesophagus.It has blind distal end with a baloon to prevent gastric aspiration. A mask at the proximal end, which can be fitted over the face. Oxygen or air can be administered through this which will come out of the holes present at the pharyngolaryngeal portion of the tube (Fig. 16.8).

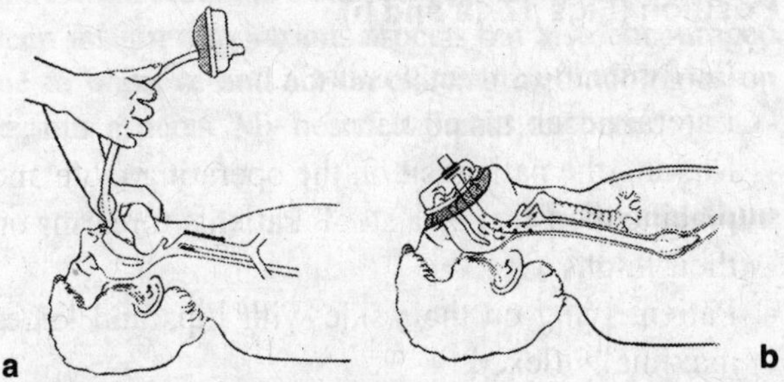

Fig. 16.8: **a.** Esophageal obturator airway-insertion and **b.** in position

17

Regional Anaesthetic Techniques (Conduction Block)

A. Equipments required for regional techniques:
   1. Spinal needle-for spinal block (Subarachnoid block, spinal anaesthesia).
   2. Epidural needle-for epidural block (Epidural anaesthesia).
   3. Double inflatable cuff with manometer for Bier's block (Regional intravenous anaesthesia).
   4. Teflon catheters.
   5. Nerve stimulator.
   6. Cleaning tray.
   7. Iodine/spirit.
   8. Sterile towel/drapes/gowns/gloves.
   9. Sterile dressings.
   10. Adhesives.

B. Resuscitation cart should be available.

C. Written consent to be taken for any technique.

SPINAL ANAESTHESIA

Objective: To provide anaesthesia for procedures and surgeries (like urological, gynaecological, obstetrical, surgical and orthopaedic cases) by giving local anaesthetics into the subarachnoid space.

Position (Figs 17.1a and b)

- Performed in sitting posture. Or
- Lateral decubitus position.
- Making the patient sit on the operating table and placing their feet on a stool. Patients forearms on their thighs. Or
- Patient lying on their side with hips and knees maximally flexed.

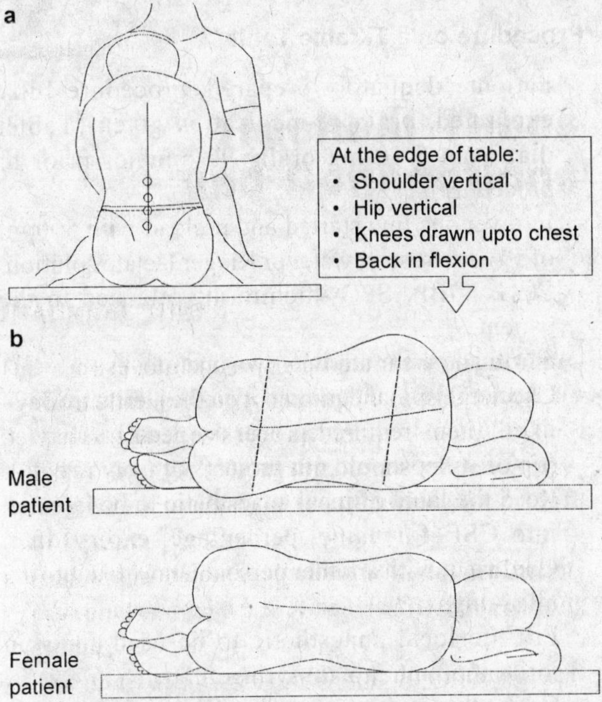

Figs 17.1a and b: Positions for spinal block

- Assistant stands in front of the patient to help in maintaining the patient in a comfortable curled position (rolled like a ball).
- The main aim of proper positioning is to obtain maximum flexion of the lumbar spine (Fig. 17.2).

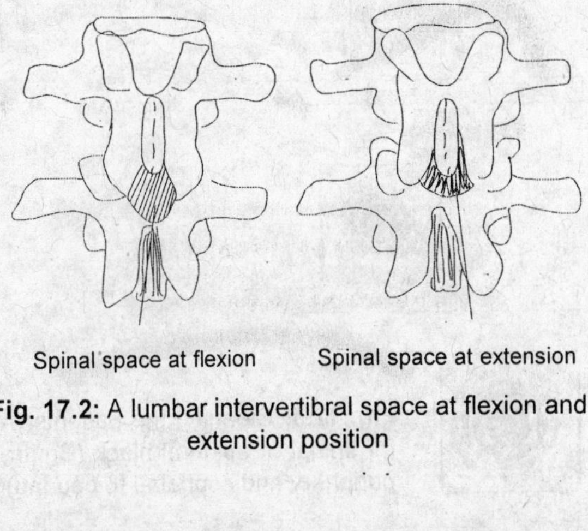

Fig. 17.2: A lumbar intervertibral space at flexion and extension position

Procedure on a Tiltable Table

- Patient adequately prepared, procedure fully explained, oral pre-medication given (Tablet diazepam 5-10 mg orally 90 minutes prior to procedure).
- Intravenous line started and preload with 500 ml of 5% dextrose in water or Ringer lactate solution.
- ECG, NIBP, SPO_2-monitoring attached to the patient.
- Scrub and wear sterile gown and gloves.
- Check the spinal equipment on the sterile trolley–like the items required: proper size needle and stylet, (tip of stylet should not project out from needle).
- Read the label of local anaesthetic to be injected into CSF–for name, percentage, expiry date. Confirm it with another person. Draw this into a 5 ml syringe.
- Fill the local anaesthetic to be used for skin infiltration into a 2 ml syringe.
- Cover the drug tray with sterile towel to avoid contamination during cleaning.
- Clean the patients back with antiseptic swabs (savalon, iodine and spirit).
- Swab eliptically from the proposed site radially outwards: cephalad to caudal direction (Fig. 17.3).

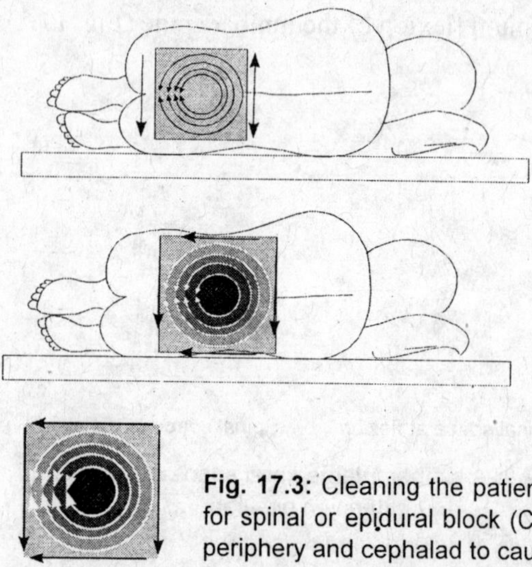

Fig. 17.3: Cleaning the patients back for spinal or epidural block (Centre to periphery and cephalad to caudad)

- Detergents to be kept outside the sterile injection tray to avoid accidental mix-up.
- Sufficiently large area is cleaned.
- Allow the iodine to dry on the skin.
- If the glove is smeared with antiseptic, change them.
- Drape the area with sterile towels.
- Highest point of iliac crest palpated and corresponding level (L_4) space is located (Fig. 17.4).

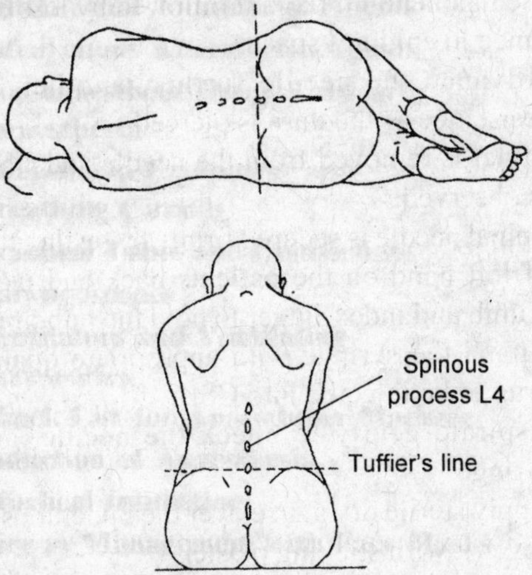

Figure: 17.4

- At the proposed L_4 space, raise an intradermal wheal with local anaesthetic with a disposable 25 G needle.
- Spinal needles are 8-10 cm long and each needle is provided with a stylet.
- The distal end of spinal needle is specialised and short bevelled to avoid post dural puncture headache (Fig. 17.5).

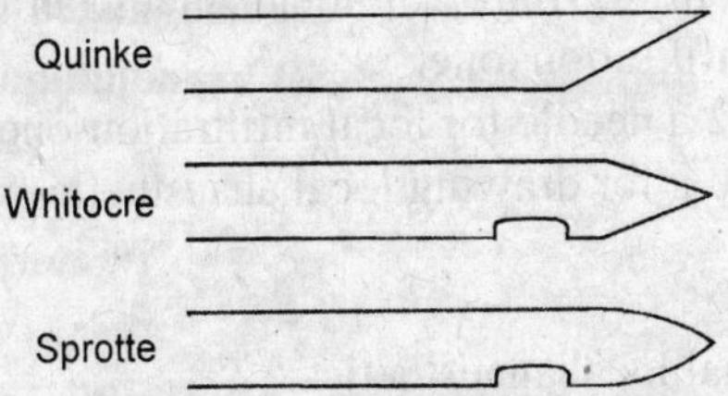

Fig. 17.5: Tip design of spinal needles

- The size varies from 20 G to 26 G.
- Thin needles are difficult to insert, so introducer is used.
- Introducers are short length, thick needle with or without flange.
- Insert the introducer if using a thin 24-25 gauge needle up to interspinous ligament.
- Insert the spinal needle through the introducer into the space.
- Increased resistance will be felt as the needle enters the ligamendum flavum followed by loss of resistance in epidural space.
- Advance the needle further, another loss of resistance as the dura is pierced.
- Stylet is removed from the needle and CSF flow is observed.
- Spinal needle is secured firmly by resting the back of left hand on the patients back and using the thumb and index finger to hold the hub of needle.
- Attach the syringe with appropriate quantity of drug to be injected into CSF.
- Aspirate gently to check the needle, and the syringe.
- Apply sterile dry gauze over the puncture site and cover it with sticking plaster.
- Patient placed supine on the table as quick as possible, may flex hips onto abdomen.
- Onset of action within few seconds.

Equipments Required for Spinal Block

A. Autoclaved or disposable presterilized items.
- Spinal needle–ideal 24-25 gauge needle–one each.
- Spinal needle introducer-one.
- 5 ml syringe for spinal anaesthetic solution–one.
- 2 ml syringe for local anaesthetic for skin infiltration–one.
- 22 g needle for local infiltration-one.
- 20 g for drawing local anaesthetic-two.

Drugs

A. Spinal local anaesthetics:

1. Lignocaine 5% heavy (hyperbaric).
2. Bupivacaine (Marcaine) 0.5% heavy, (hyperbaric) (sensorcaine).
3. Cinchocaine (Nupercaine, Dibucaine) 0.5%, heavy (hyperbaric).
4. Amethocaine (Tetracaine, Pintocaine, Pontocaine, Decicain, Butethanol, Anethaine) 1% solution prepared in saline, water or dextrose.
5. Mepivacaine (Scandicaine, Carbocaine, Meaverin)–4%, heavy (hyperbaric)

B. Vasopressors: Metaraminol (Aramine)
- Ephedrine
- Methoamine (Vasoxine)
- Phenylephrine
- Noradrenaline/adrenaline
- Mephentermine.

C. Sterile Cutting File: Sterile drapes-Four separate towels or a single sheet with centre eye hole.
D. Resusciatation equipment
E. Cleaning Tray-Gallipot, sponge holding forceps, sterile gauze swabs.
F. Antiseptic–savalon, iodine, spirit.
G. Intravenous Cannula–18 G/16 G
H. Intravenous infusion set and intravenous fluids
- 5% Dextrose
- Normal Saline
- Ringer's lactate
- Haemaccel.

I. Patient monitors-ECG, SPO_2, NIBP.

Important Points

Complete asepsis is observed:
- Drugs checked before given and no multi dose vials should be used for spinal.
- Resuscitation equipments always ready (Table 17.1).
- Maintain silence in the operating room during regional technique.
- The degree of spinal block is achieved by positioning the patient after the drug is given in the subarachnoid space–like

1. Upper abdominal-level required
   - Surgery-T_4–T_5 (Nipple level)
2. Lower abdominal-T_6–T_8 (Xiphi–sternum) (Caesarean section, hernia, etc).
3. Prostatic, Vaginal surgery, hip surgery etc–T_{10} (Umbilicus)
4. Lower limb surgery-L_1 (Groin)
5. Perineal and rectal surgery-S_2 (Perineum)

Table 17.1: Things required for Resuscitation cart

- Anaesthesia machine with breathing circuit/Manual resuscitator.
- Oxygen source attached to the machine (Cylinder or pipeline)
- Equipment required for tracheal intubation (as mentioned earlier)
- Suction apparatus
- Emergency drugs:
  a. Vasopressors–Adrenline, Noradrenaline, Dopamine. Dobutamine, Metaraminol, Methoxamine, Mephentermine, Phenylerphrine.
  b. Antihypertensive–Nifedepin, Isoptin, Nitroprusside, Nitroglycerine.
  c. Sodium Bicarbonate, calcium chloride.
  d. Hydrocortisone, Dexamethazone.
  e. Aminophylline.
  f. Antihistamines-Pheniramine.
  g. Antiemetic-Stemetil, Siquil, Droperidol.
  h. Antiarrhythmic–Xylocard, Isoptin, Procainamide, Propranolol, amiodorone.
  i. Atropine Sulphate.
  j. Anticonvulsants-Diazepam, Dilantin sodium, Thiopentone.
- Intravenous Fluids-Crystalloids and Colloids and infusion sets.
- Disposable Syringes (2, 5, 10, 20, 50 ml) and needles (16, 18, 20, 22 G), IV canula (16, 18, 20 G) and three ways.
- Defibrillator.

Spinal Anaesthesia in Obstetrics

Objective: To provide anaesthesia for caesarean section, manual removal of placenta or repair of third degree perineal tear.

Position

Lateral position is favoured (as described earlier).

Procedure: Procedure same as in non pregnant patients (described earlier). Pregnant women need smaller volumes of anaesthetic solution.

- Bupivacaine 2 to 2.5 ml.5%, hyperbaric solution.
- Bupivacaine 2 to 2.5 ml 0.5 %, Isobaric solution.
- Lignocaine 1.4 to 1.6 ml 5 %, hyperbaric solution. (Lignocaine with adrenaline 0.2 ml of 1 : 1000) 2 to 2.5 ml 2%, Isobaric solution.
- Lignocaine 0.9 ml 5%, hyperbaric solution (for forceps delivery).
- Lignocaine 1.5 ml 5%, hyperbaric solution (For manual removal of placenta).

Equipments Required

Same as described earlier.

EPIDURAL ANAESTEHSIA

Objective

To provide anaesthesia for procedures and surgeries like urological, gynaecological, obstetrics, abdominal and orthopaedic surgeries by giving anaesthetics into the epidural space. Epidural space is between the ligamentom flavum and durameter.

This technique is also used for providing post-operative analgesia.

Written consent for procedure required.

Position

Same as for spinal required.

Procedure

On a tiltable table.

- Procedure explained to the patient.
- Oral premedication given.
- Performed at any level of spinal cord according to the desired level of analgesia.
- Thoracic, lumber or caudal epidural practiced.
- Needle insertion in each region is different because of the anatomy of the spine.
- The duration of action can be prolonged by intermittent injections through an epidural catheter.

- Epidural needles are thick, and curved tips (16, 18, 20 G tuohy) (Figs 17.6 and 17.7).

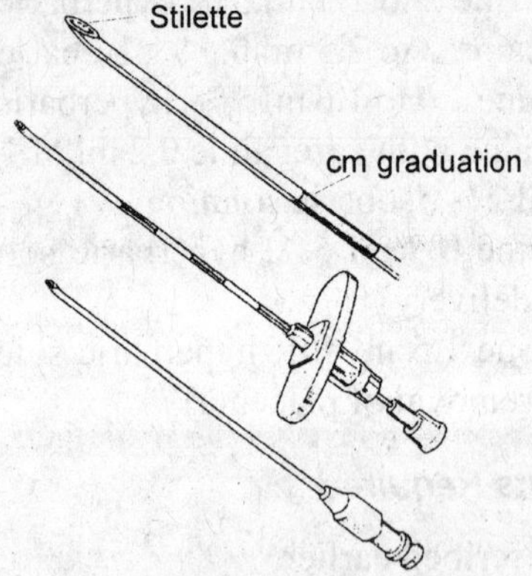

Fig. 17.6: Epidural needles

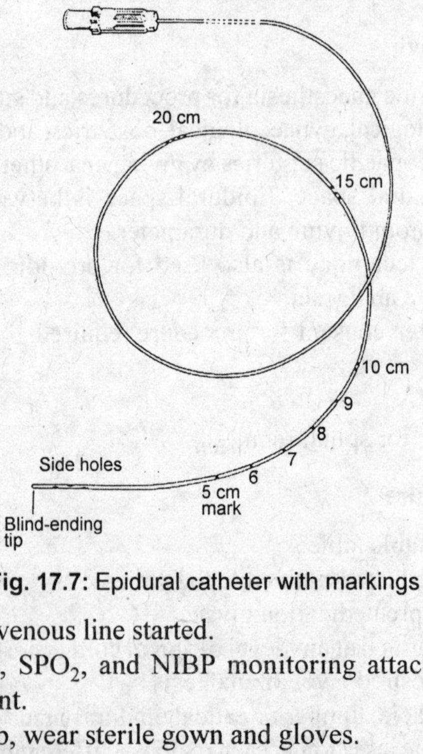

Fig. 17.7: Epidural catheter with markings

- Intravenous line started.
- ECG, SPO_2, and NIBP monitoring attached to patient.
- Scrub, wear sterile gown and gloves.
- Check the epidural set on the sterile trolley for the items required, proper size needle and catheter, proper fitting of syringe into the hub of epidural needle.

- Fill in a 20 ml syringe the local anaesthetic to be injected into the epidural space.
- Read the label of drug vial carefully for the name, percentage, baricity, expiry date. Confirm it with your assistant.
- Fill the local anaesthetic to be used for skin infiltration into a 2 ml syringe (2 cc, 2% xylocaine).
- Cover the drug tray with a sterile towel. To avoid spilling of antiseptic solution during cleaning.
- Clean the back with anticeptic swab same as spinal procedure.
- At L_4 space, skin is infilterated with local anaesthesia with a 24/25 G needle.
- A skin puncture is made with a 18G needle.
- Epidural needle is introduced in the above point upto supraspinous ligament.
- Stylet is withdrawn and attach a 10 ml syringe with 5-6 ml of air.
- Needle is advanced further using firm but gentle pressure on the plunger of the syringe till there is a sudden loss of resistance to pressure on the plunger.
- The epidural space correct position is further checked by adding a drop of local anaesthetic deposited at the hub which will be sucked in.
- The drug slowly injected attaching the 20 ml syringe into the epidural space, directly after a test dose of 2 ml or
- Epidural catheter is inserted through the needle, if intermittent dosage is required.
- The catheter is introduced up to 3rd mark.
- Needle is carefully withdrawn.
- Catheter is adjusted up to 2nd mark
- It is fixed to the back of the patient.
- Drug is given through the catheter slowly.
- Onset of action after 15-20 minutes.

Equipments Required for Epidural

A. Autoclaved or disposable presterilized items.
  - Epidural needle.
  - Epidural catheter/with or without a filter.

- 10 ml syringe for testing-one
- 5 ml syringe for local infiltration–one
- 20 ml syringe for epidural drug–one
- 18 G needle for skin puncture–one
- 20 G needle for drug aspiration–one
- 22 G needle for skin infiltration–one.

B. Drugs
1. 2% xylocane plain/with adrenaline
   0.5 % Bupivacaine plain
2. Vasopressors.

C. Cleaning Tray
D. Antiseptics
E. Sterile drapes
F. Resuscitation equipments
G. Intravenous canula-18 G/16G
H. Intravenous infusion sets and IV fluids
I. Patient monitor-ECG, SPO_2, NIBP.

Approximate volume required for epidural block: (Lignocaine hydrochloride–1.5% solution)

- Suprapubic Prostatectomy-10-30 ml
- Vaginal and Perineal repair-20-35 ml
- Hernia appendectomy-20-30 ml
- Upper abdomen operations-35-40 ml
- Caesarean section-15-20 ml
  - 35 mg/spinal segment
  - 15 mg/spinal segment (old age)

Bupivacaine:

- Maximum safe dose-2 ml/kg (25-30 ml 0.5% solution)
- 0.75 % more profound effect
- 0.25 % post operative pain relief.
- Average lower laparotomies-15-25 ml (0.5%)
- Average upper laparotomies–30 ml (0.5%).

Thoracic Epidurals

Objective: To provide segmental analgesia for operation and pain relief in the thoracic region by introducing local anaesthetics or narcotics into the epidural space.

Position: Sitting or lateral position as for spinal described earlier.

Procedure: Same as that of lumbar epidural except that the procedure is performed in the thoracic region and technique of needle insertion is:

i. Skin puncture is just lateral to the spinous process at the inferior aspect of the interspace.
ii. Needle directed 10° medially and 45° cephalad.

Equipment required for thoracic epidural: same as that of lumbar epidural.

Volume required:

i. 1.5% lignocaine or 0.5% bupivacaine 3 to 5 ml for a block of 2-4 segments.
ii. For constant infusion-0.125% bupivacaine 10-15 ml/hour for postoperative analgesia.

Caudal Block

Objective: To provide anaesthesia and analgesia for perineal, pelvic and abdominal operations by introducing the local anaesthetic or opiod analgesic into the caudal epidural space.

Position (Fig. 17.8):

- Lateral position, or
- Prone position with hips slightly flexed over two pillows. Legs slightly abducted and toes turn in.
- Knee chest position.
- Knee elbow position.

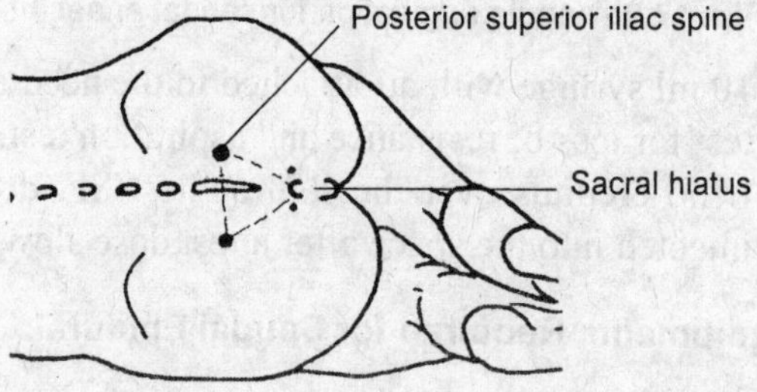

Fig. 17.8: Patient position for caudal anaesthesia (lateral)

Procedure:

- Patient is premedicated with oral drugs.
- Intravenous line secured.
- In children–under light general anaesthesia (with O_2, N_2O halothane).
- Clean the lower back.

- Drape the part with sterile towels leaving the sacrococcygeal region exposed.
- Tip of coccyx identified.
- Triangular sacral hiatus palpated, 3.5-5 cm above it.
- Local infiltration usually not given (to preserve landmarks).
- 5 cm needle, 22 g is inserted through the sacro-cocygeal membrane at an angle of 20° (No need to use epidural needle). Once through the membrane, the needle is depressed to further 45° towards the intergluteal cleft and the needle is advanced further 2-3 cm in the midline. The needle should not go beyond the level of post inferior iliac spine (Fig. 17.9).

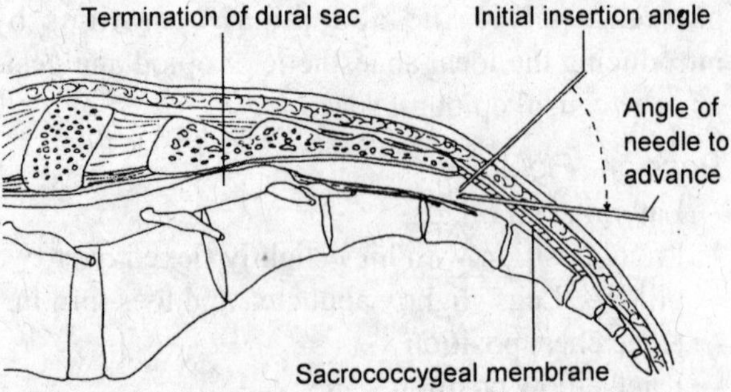

Fig. 17.9: Needle angulation for caudal anaesthesia

- 10 ml syringe with air attached to the needle and test for loss of resistance and aspiration test.
- If no crepitus over the skin or no CSF, drug is injected into the space after a test dose slowly.

Equipments Required for Caudal Epidural

Same as lumbar epidural.

Volume Required

Operations on anus, rectum, perineum or urethra, (circumcision, vagino-plasty etc.)

(Up to L_2-L_4)–lignacaine 1-2 % with or without adrenaline, bupivacaine 0.25–0.5% 10-30 ml.

- For post operative analgesia–30 ugm per kilogram body weight morphine sulphate diluted in 10-15 ml of normal saline solution.
- For infants and children–analgesia supplemented with light general anaesthesia for operations and procedures and for post operative analgesia.

Recommended Doses

Bupivacaine Plain: 0.5 % solution, 0.5 ml/year age

Or 1.5 mg/kg 0.25% solution 1 ml/year of age.

Or 0.5-1.25 mg/kg.

Lignocaine with adrenaline: 1% solution 1 ml/year of age.

Or 1 ml/dermatome per year of age (Upper limit 6 mg per kg).

Nerve Blocks

Nerve block comprises an injection of a local anaesthetics to a peripheral or central sensory nerve, plexus or sympathetic plexus. It is used to alleviate pain during operation, post operative period or in chronic pain conditions.

Things required are:

- Cleaning tray, savalon, iodine, sprit
- Sterile drapes, towels
- Syringes, needles
- Local anaesthetics
- Nerve stimulator
- Sterile dressings and adhesives

Any regional blocks, resuscitation kit should be ready for emergency need and written consent to be taken.

18

Monitoring During Anaesthesia

A. Monitoring Electrical Cardiac Activity (ECG)

Objective

To monitor electrical cardiac activity for all anaesthetized and sick non anaesthetized patients. Monitoring ECG helps in detection of cardiac dysrhythmias and ischaemia.

Technique

1. The ECG electrodes (RA, LA and LL), RA and LA over the right and left upper chest or shoulder and LL at the apex or CM5 lead configuration (Fig. 18.1).

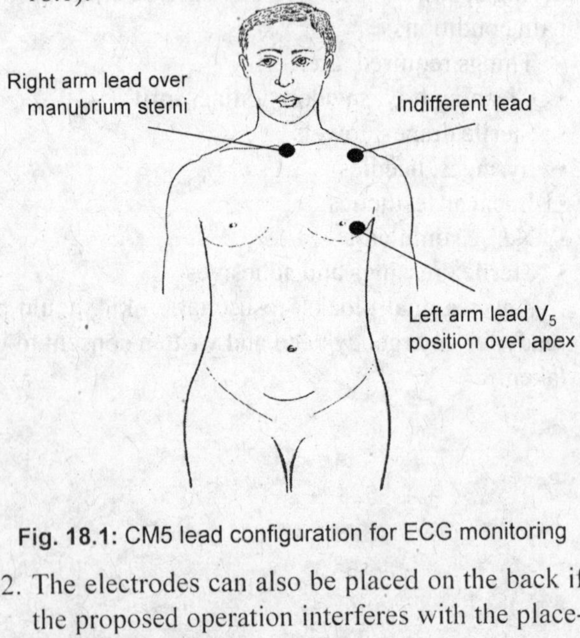

Fig. 18.1: CM5 lead configuration for ECG monitoring

2. The electrodes can also be placed on the back if the proposed operation interferes with the placement of electrodes.

3. If the surgeons hands or procedures interferes, the placement should be done slightly above or below accordingly.
4. The ECG monitor cables are attached to the electrodes.
5. The monitor is earthed properly.
6. The machine is put on; upper and lower limit alarms are set; machine is adjusted to L II system.

Equipments Required

1. ECG monitor (3 lead or 5 lead system).
2. ECG electrodes.
3. Electrode jelly.

Equipment care and precautions:

1. The machine should be placed properly on a trolley or table.
2. The earth wire is properly attached.
3. Before shifting the patient from the O.T. table, the ECG cables are disconnected.
4. The cables are cleaned with gauze, coiled and kept for next use.

B. Blood Pressure Monitoring (Non-invasive)

Objective

Mechanical cardiac activity can be assessed by arterial blood pressure observations.

Technique

a. Manually operated
   1. Place the stethoscope diaphragm over the brachial artery just above the bend in the elbow or on the medial side of the arm and secured to the arm by fastening the holding strap snugly.
   2. The BP cuff is applied in such a way that the rubber inflatable bag is over the artery. Winding is firm but not tight.
   3. Cuff is inflated to a level about 20 mmHg above the anticipated systolic blood pressure. Pressure is reduced 2 mm Hg per sec while auscultating over the arterial site.

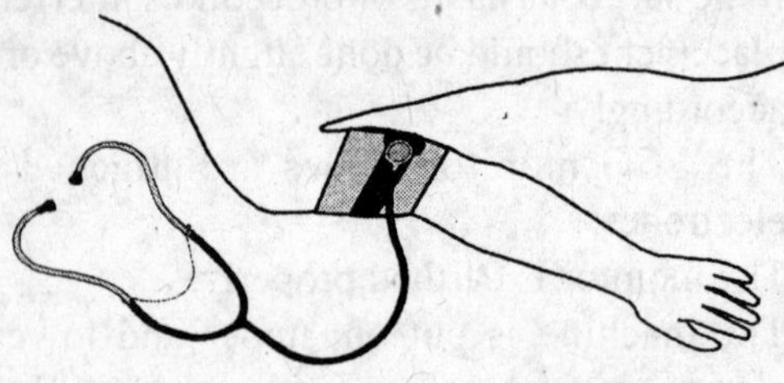

Fig. 18.2: Application of stethoscope

Equipments required:

1. Sphygmomanometer and different sizes cuff or Aneroid manometer.

Standard bladder sizes and lengths (American Heart Association)

a. Mercury manometer
b. Compression Bag–20% wider than the diameter of the arm

	Width (cm)	*Length cm*
Obese adult	18-20	30-35
Adult's thigh	18	35
Adult's arm	12.5	35
4-10 yrs	9.5	23
1-4 yrs	6	15
infant (1 yr)	4	12
New born (< 1 month)	2.5	5

2. Stethoscope without bell on diaphragm. Length of the tubing to be adequate enough to reach the anaesthetist's ears without bending.

b. Blood pressure monitoring by automatic method:
   1. Equipment–Automated Oscillometers.
   2. No need to fix the stethoscope.
   3. The cuff is tied on the arm or thigh.
   4. The machine is switched on; and adjusted for the time interval at which the readings are required.

C. Venous Pressure Monitoring (CVP)

Objective: The venus pressure is measured at the junction of right atrium and the venacavae. CVP canulation is an aid for fluid management, use of ionotropes, for repeated blood sampling and administration of parental nutrition.

Technique: Sites are chosen according to the suitability of site and requirement. Commonly used sites are Basilic, and, internal jugular vein).

Position

1. Patient Supine, head turned to the opposite side; pillow under the shoulder; patient placed slightly in the trendelenberg position.
2. Land Mark–Sternomastoid muscle sternal head and clavicular head makes triangle, the apex of the triagle denotes the point of puncture (Fig. 18.3).

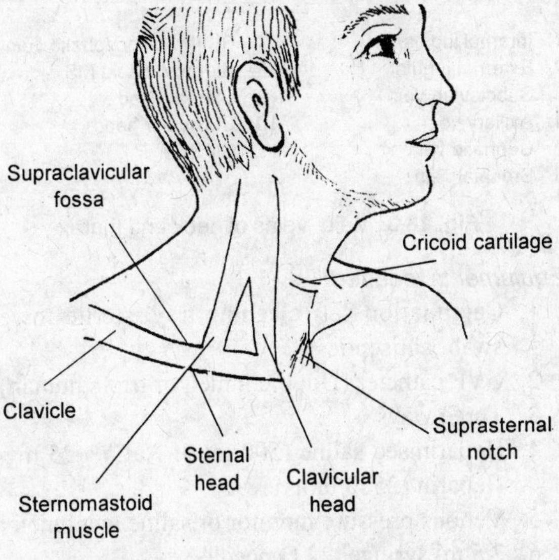

Fig. 18.3: Landmarks used in Int. Jugular cannulations

3. 22 gauge needle attached to a 5 ml syringe with 2 ml heparinised saline is inserted at 45° to the skin at this point, aiming at the nipple or hip. Once the vein is identified the needle is removed. At the same location as before cannula with stillete inserted confirm after aspirating blood, the stillete is removed and the 'j' wire is introduced and the catheter is withdrawn. A no 11 scalpel blade is used to widen the puncture site. Venous dilator is inserted over the wire into the vein upto the hub and the dilator withdrawn. The CVP catheter is

threaded through this wire and the wire withdrawn (Fig. 18.4).

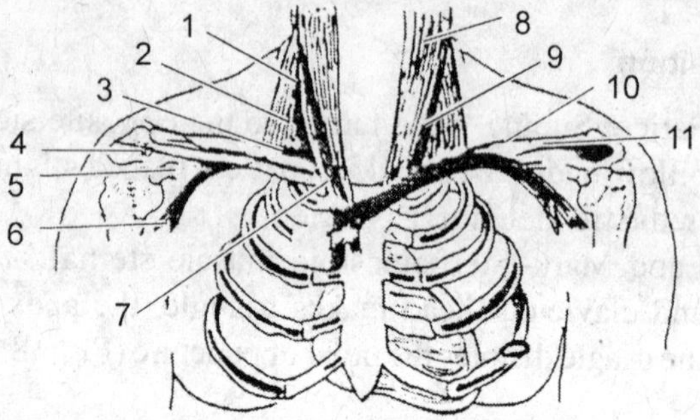

1. Internal jugular
2. External jugular
3. Subclavian vein
4. Axillary vein
5. Cephalic vein
6. Brachial vein
7. Rt. brachiocephalic vein
8. Sternomastoid MS
9. Sternal head
10. Clavicular head
11. Clavicle

Fig. 18.3: Major veins of neck and thorax

Equipments required:

1. Cannulation set (cleaning tray, sterile towels, swab, antiseptics)
2. CVP catheter (Double lumen or triple human)
3. Three ways
4. Heparinised saline (500 ml of NaCl + 25 mg of Heparin (2500 units)
5. Venous pressure monitor or saline manometer.
6. 2,5 ml syringe, 22 G needle
7. Leveller
8. Scale/adhesives/dressings
9. Extension tubing (70 cm length).

Precautions: The transducer diaphragm is very sensitive to proteinous substances. It should not be contaminated with blood. Avoid backflow of blood Vigilant sterile precautions should be used.

D. Direct Arterial Blood Pressure Monitoring

Objective: To measure the arterial blood presure directly by introducing an indwelling catheter into any palpable artery, commonly used is radial artery.

Technique

1. Non dominant hand, radial artery preferred.
2. The wrist dorsiflexed (Figs 18.5 and 18.6), immobilized, cleaned with iodine and spirit prior to catheter insertion.

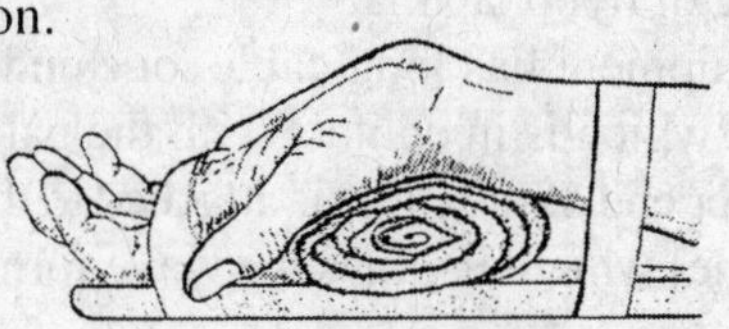

Fig. 18.5: Position for arterial cannulation

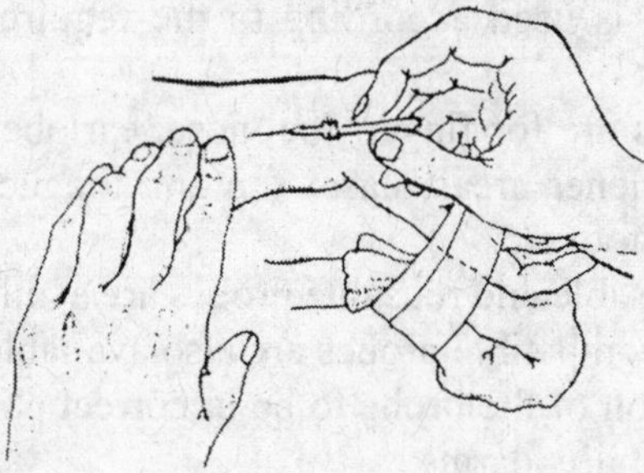

Fig. 18.6: Insertion of arterial catheter in Radial artery

3. 20 G cannula is used.
4. Palpate the artery with left hand index and middle finger and the needle and catheter introduced through the skin into the artery. Once the artery is punctured, the needle is withdrawn and the distal end of cannula attached to an extension line filled with heparinised saline.
5. The arterial cannula is fixed properly with adhesive. The joints are tightened. If cannula with port, it is sealed to avoid any accidental injections of drugs.

Equipments:

1. Intra arterial Pressure monitor
2. Transducer cable
3. 3 ways–Three

D. Pulse Oximetry

- Pulse oximetry is a non-invasive method of measuring oxygen saturation (SpO_2).

- It is measures continuously.
- It also provides a continuous pulse rate and beat to beat monitoring of the peripheral pulse.
- The main purpose of pulse oximetry is to provide warning of hypoxaemia.
- The equipment has long cable, one end, a sensor (Probe) which is in contact with the patient.
- The other end of the cable is attached to the console (machine) which displays the wave forms and the reading.
- Different types and sizes of probes are available which is used according to the requirement of patients.
- Probes are for finger, toe, nose, earlobe, thener, hypothener areas, nasal septum, tongue, check, palm, foot etc.
- Disposable and reusable probes are available.
- MRI compatible probes are also available.
- Fixation of the probe to be in correct position to avoid false alarms.
- Appearance of a satisfactory waveform is a good indication that the readings are reliable.
- This is used during anaesthesia, transport, ICUs, HDUs, wards.
- This is one of the essential monitoring standards used during anaesthesia.
- The distal end of the cable to be secured or tied with the hand.
- Follow manufacturer's instruction.

E. Neuro muscular Monitoring

- Neuromuscular stimulators are used to monitor the degree of neuromuscular block.
- The electrical stimulus is delivered near a peripheral motor nerve and it is evaluated by its response on the muscles innervated by that nerve.
- These stimulators are battery operated and calibrated in milli amperes (mA)and deliver the set current.
- The current suitable for stimulating nerves are between 20-60 mA for skin electrodes and 5-8 mA for needle electrodes.

- The frequency of stimuli is expressed in Hertz (HZ) which is 1 cycle/sec (0.1 Hz is equal to 1 Stimulus every 10 sec).
- Commonly used rates are 0.1 to 100 Hz.
- Stimulation is achieved by placing the electrodes along a nerve and passing current through them. It can be achieved directly, by placing surface electrodes or by needle electrodes. The negative is placed distally.

F. Temperature Monitoring

- Number of body sites are used for measuring temperature–Nasopharynx, esophagus, rectum, skin, middle ear, axilla, urinary bladder, pulmonary artery or trachea.
- Usually the nasopharyngeal or rectal temperature (the least reliable) is measured in the operation theatre.
- Temperature monitoring is a continuous process.
- The equipment used are thermistor, thermocouple, Platinum wire liquid crystal and infrared
- Disposable and reusable temperature probes are available.
- For calibration, cleaning and maintenance manufacturer's instruction to be followed.

G. Gas Monitoring

Different technologies are used to measure the inspired and end tidal concentration of O_2, nitrogen, CO_2, nitrous oxide and the volatile anaesthetic agents. Those are:

- Mass Spectrometry:
- Raman Light Scattering Gas Analysis
- Infrared Analysis
- Paramagnetic Analysis
- Piezoelectric Analysis
- Chemical methods
- Refractometry

While using these technologies accurate calibrations to be done according to manufactures guidelines and instructions.

Oxygen Monitor

- During anaesthesia O_2 in the breathing system is measured by oxygen analyzer.
- It detects low or high oxygen delivery.
- It detects disconnection in the breathing system.
- It detects hypoventilation.

Carbondioxide Monitor

- CO_2 analysis provides means for assessing ventilation.
- The sampling of the gas is taken from the breathing circuit.
- It can detect many equipment and patient related problems.
- Capnometer is used to measure CO_2 concentrations during the respiratory cycle and the respiratory rate.
- It also helps in determining the correct placement of the endotracheal or endobronchial tube,serve as a warning of accidental bronchial intubation,it can alert the anaesthetist the wearing off of the muscle relaxant.
- Many capnometers are part of multipurpose monitors with other parameters used during anaesthesia.
- It shows the wave forms as well as the digital display.
- Portable,battery operated CO_2 monitoring devices for emergency medicine and patient transport are available.
- MRI compatible CO_2 monitors are also available.

Volatile Anaesthetic agents Monitor

- Gas monitors are used for monitoring halogenated anaesthetic agents.
- It assess the voporizer function and content.
- Detects inadvertent administration.
- Information on uptake and elimination.
- Information on anaesthetic depth.
- Detects contaminants if present.

MONITORING AIRWAY PRESSURE, VOLUMES, AND FLOWS

- A respirometer displays volumetric measurements of gas-tidal volume and minute volumes.
- Monitoring respiratory volumes and flows can aid in detecting obstructions, disconnections, leaks, apnoea, ventilator failure, etc.
- Respirometers can be attached to the breathing system.
- Both adult and infant versions are available.
- Wright Respirometer, Drager volumeter, Spiromed are some of the models available.
- It can be an integral part of the anaesthesia machine or ventilator with alarms.

Airway Pressure Monitor

It warns abnormal pressure conditions in the breathing system. It is usually attached to anaesthesia machine and ventilator.

Alarm Devices

- Alarms devices are warning signals generated by equipments.
- It alerts the personnel.
- It is available in most equipments.
- It can be audio, visual or both.
- Alarm settings are to be adjusted before using the machine.

19

Positioning During Anaesthesia

POSITIONING IN ANAESTHESIA AND SURGERY

- Practical and theoretical understanding of general principles of positioning, planning for a particular surgery or procedure,operating room personnel and devices required for the positioning are the key points to safe positioning.
- If the positioning is not correct it will lead to complications.
- A full knowledge about the surgical table and its control knobs used for different operations and procedures, help during the positioning.
- Protective padding to be given at different vulnerable sites. Body points that needs padding are:
  - Occipital padding for–supine position;
  - Eye and ear padding for–lateral positioning;
  - Elbow and its cubital area padding for–dorsal and lateral decubitus position, and pronated with arms along side the hand position.
  - Knees padding for—kneeling prone position;
  - Any of the dorsal decubitus position–heels to be padded.
- If the positioning is not correct, it can lead to:
  - Eye injury,
  - Nerve injury,
  - Soft tissue injury,
  - Respiratory, circulatory, central nervous complications,
  - Visceral damage, and
  - Deliterious physiological changes.

- Different procedures demand specific positions. Thus we have,

Supine	Lithotomy
Prone	Trendelenberg
Lateral (Rt./Lt.)	Fowlers
Jack-knife	Knee-elbow
Sitting	Knee-chest
	Kidney-bridge

Overholt's and Parry Brown positions.

20

Infection Control and Aseptic Practices

INFECTION CONTROL

- During anaesthesia and surgery there is an increased risk of developing infections.
- Strict infection control practices to be followed.
- All items used for the patient should be sterile.
- For all invasive and non-invasive procedures, proper infection control practices to be followed.
- The most important infection control practice to be observed is hand washing before and after procedures.
- Select appropriate barrier precautions.
- Avoid any injury during working.
- No recapping of needles.
- Segregation of waste and disposal to be followed according to the hospital protocol.

Aseptic Practices

Objectives: To reduce endogenous, and exogenous, source of infections to patients and health care workers.

Types of Aseptic practices:

- Hand Washing.
- Use of Sterilized equipments, machines and articles.
- Use of barrier nursing.
- Adopting universal and barrier precautions.
- Care of indwelling devices.
- Proper decontamination and Sterilization of equipments.
- Isolation of infected from clean/non infected.
- Environmental cleaning, hygiene, sterilisation.
- Proper disposal of hospital waste.

Indications

Patient:
- During Surgical procedures, endoscopic techniques, and procedures.
- During care and nursing of patients.
- During intravascular access and procedures.
- During invasive and non-invasive monitoring.
- During diagnostic and therapeutic procedures.

Equipments:
During decontamination and sterilization.

Hospital and environment:
During cleaning, decontamination and waste disposal.

Hand Washing

Objective: To Decontaminate the hands to prevent transfer of infection from hands to patients

- **Organism Responsible for spread of infection through hands:** Coagulase negative Staphylococci, diphtheroids, Candida (natural flora which survive and multiply in the skin of hands) Contaminants from infected patients, environment, infected equipments and articles etc. (Transient flora can be any pathogenic organisms).
- **Types of Hand Washing:**
  - Surgical hand washing
  - Hygienic hand washing
  - Social hand washing

  Hands should be washed with soap and water.
- Before touching the patient
- After touching the patient
- Before any procedure
- After any procedure
- Before and after handling the food and drinks
- After handling equipment contaminated with body fluids and blood
- After contact with blood and body fluids
- After handling clinical waste and used laundry
- After removing gloves
- After using the toilet

- Before leaving the clinical area
- Before and after caring of immunocompromised patients.
- Before and after blood sampling, specimen handling
- **Agents used:**
- Plain water and soap
- Antiseptic detergents
  - 4% chlorhexidine
  - Povidone–iodine
  - 0.5% Chlorhexiduce
  - Povidone iodine in 70% isopropanol or ethanol.

***Steps of Handwashing: (Fig. 20.1)**

1. Wash hands with soap and water.
2. Take soap solution.
3. Rub palm to palm.
4. Right palm over the left dorsum.
5. Left palm over the right dorsum.
6. Fingers interlace palm to palm.
7. Back of fingers to opposing palms.
8. Rotational rubbing of thumbs.
9. Rotational rubbing of palms.

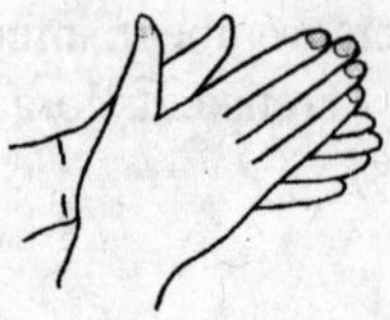

Palm to palm

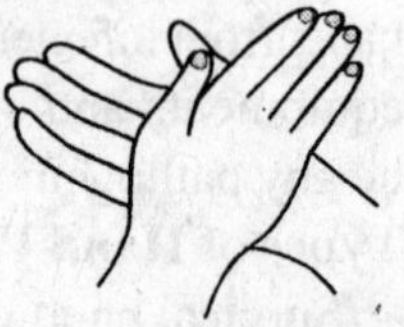

Right palm over left dorsum

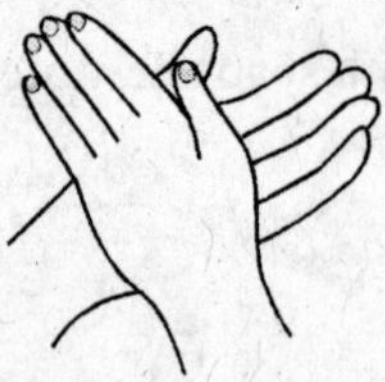

Left palm over right dorsum

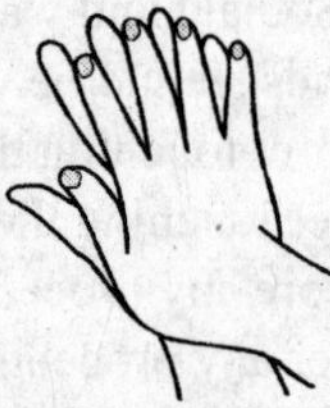

Fingers interlace palm to palm

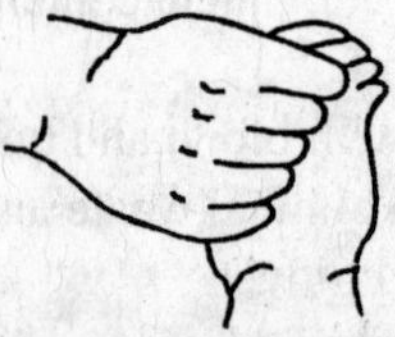

Back of fingers to opposing palms

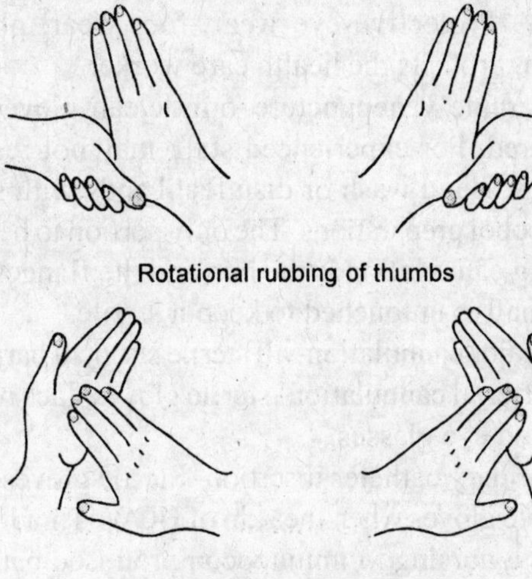

Rotational rubbing of thumbs

Rotational rubbing of palms

Fig. 20.1: Steps in hand washing

Cuts and Wounds

Damaged skin of HCW should be protected (especially hands and forearms) with dressing/waterproof dressing.

Avoid direct contact with patient, blood and body fluids.

Standard blood and body fluid precautions: It should be practiced routinely in the care of all patients regardless of whether they are known to have an infection or not.

- Maintain integrity of skin.
- Use of Protective apparels and clothing appropriately.

Barrier (According to the Type of Procedure)

Objectives: To keep a barrier between infected and non infected, or sterile and unsterile area (to prevent infection).

Barriers: For patient and HCW (Health Care Worker).

- For operations full sterile barrier precautions to be used. Use of sterile Gown, gloves, face mask, Cap-this protects infection to both patient and

HCW. Protective eye wear, foot wear, plastic apron, protects the health care worker.

- For simple venepuncture–only clean gloves are required. For experienced staff–may not require gloves. Hand wash or disinfect hands with spirit or alcohol preparations. The only portion to be held during cannulation is the hub and the flanges and the shaft is untouched to keep it sterile.
- For major cannulation–all sterile surgical barriers.
- For arterial cannulation–sterile gloves, face mask, cap and eye glasses.
- For urinary catheter insertion–Sterile gloves.
- Double gloves when the skin of HCW is not intact.
- During nursing to immunocompromised patients all surgical barriers with barrier nursing.
- During general nursing–face mask, gloves, plastic apron.
- During suctioning–(Tracheal)–sterile gloves, face mask, protective eye wear.
- Blood sampling–clean gloves.
- ICU/OT cleaning–thick rubber gloves, foot wear.
- To protect aerosol infection–face mask and eye wear (to both HCW and to patients).
- Vaginal delivery–all surgical barriers including foot wear especially gum boots.
- Specimens and sample handling–gloves.
- Blood bank staff–gloves.
- Laundary–gloves, face mask, foot wear, plastic apron and eye wear.
- Laboratory–face mask, gloves and eye wear.
- Direct pippetting avoided. Discarded specimens as hospital waste management protocol (disinfection and disposal).
- Dental procedures–mask, gloves and eye wear.
- Autopsy and embalming–Thick gloves, face mask, eye wear, foot wear and plastic apron.

During Resuscitation

- Full infection control practices should to be followed as far as possible even during in an emergency.

- It is recommended to use mouth pieces, ambu bags, airways, oesophageal obturator, LMA etc for resuscitation. These items should be disposable or resterilized properly.

Blood and Body Fluid Spills

- Spills should be avoided as far as possible.
- If accidental spill occurs, it should be removed with a detergent soaked cotton or gauze (sodium hypo chlorite solution) with a gloved hand. The material to be disposed of in the container identified as infectious Waste.

Safe Handling of Sharps

- Sharps are—Needles, scalpels, broken glass pieces coverings of bottles and vials and any item which may injure the hand.
- Careful handling of sharps.
- DO NOT RECAP needles (Fig. 20.2).

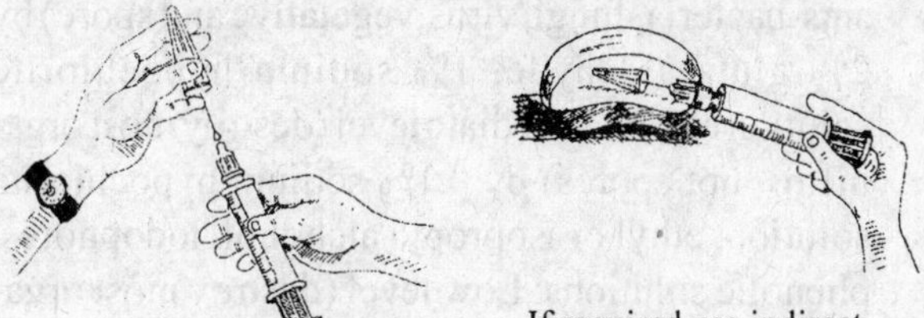

Do not recap needle — If required use indirect method

Fig. 20.2

- Immediate disposal of used sharps in appropriate puncture proof container.
- One should not carry used sharps by hand or pass to another person.
- Accidental injury with sharps–encourgage bleeding, wash immediately thoroughly with soap and water and cover with a dressing.
- Report to the hospital authority.
- If blood and body fluid splash—wash and rinse thoroughly with plenty of water.

21 Sterilisation, Disinfection, Decontamination and Biomedical Waste Management

STERILISATION, DISINFECTION AND DECONTAMINATION

- Decontamination includes cleaning, disinfecting and sterilising.
- Sterilisation is the process of destroying all micro-organisms including spores; e.g. steam, dry heat, ETO.
- Disinfection is the process of decontamination by various types: high level (destroy all micro-organisms-bacteria, fungi, virus;vegetative and spore) by 2% glutaraldehyde, 1% sodium hypochlorite solution etc; Intermediate level (destroy most organisms, not spores) by 0.1% sodium hypochlorite solution, ethyl or isopropyl alchohol, iodophores, phenolic solutions; Low level (destroy most organisms, not spores and non enveloped virus, mycobacteria) by quaternary ammonium compounds like savalon, dettol etc.
- Recommendations for sterilisation and disinfection:
  - *Airways and endotracheal tubes:* autoclave or chemical disinfection;as far as possible use disposables.
  - *Laryngoscope:* blade after use, clean with water and soap/detergent (70% isopropyl alcohol). Handle, clean it with alcohol and wet cloth; store in a dry sterile linen.
  - *Surgical instruments:* after cleaning, autoclave.
  - *Flexible and rigid endoscopes:* all channels flush and clean with water and brushed;

channels rinsed with high level disinfectant followed by sterile water and 70% alcohol always follow manufacturer's instructions.

- *Stethoscope:* wipe with 70% alcohol.
- *BP cuffs:* clean with 70% alcohol or wash with soap and water if soiled.
- *Anaesthesia circuits* (non disposables) wash with running water and immerse in 2% glutaraldehyde for 30 minutes, rinse with water and dry.
- *Face mask:* wash with water and soap/2% gluteraldehyde.
- *Pulse oximeter probe/temperature probe:* disinfect with 70% alcohol.
- Sterile disposable items to be used for invasive and semi invasive procedures.

BIOMEDICAL WASTE MANAGEMENT (BMW)

- Proper hospital waste management to followed at all times.
- It is very important to prevent infection to patient, from patient to health care workers and patient to patient.
- Categorisation of BMW:
  - Category-1 : Human Anatomical Waste.
  - Category-2 : Animal Waste
  - Category-3 : Microbiology and Biotechnology Waste
  - Category-4 : Sharps
  - Category-5 : Discarded Medicines and Cytotoxic Waste
  - Category-6 : Solid Waste (plaster casts and Bandages Soiled with Blood and Body Secretions)
  - Category-7 : Plastics and Disposables
  - Category-8 : Liquid Waste
  - Category-9 : Incinerator Ash
  - Category-10 : Chemical Waste

- Seggregation, Transportation, Pre-treatement, Treatment and Final disposal should be done according to the protocol laid by the hospital.
- Strictly one should follow the hospital policies and guidelines to safeguard the safety of operation theatre personnel during BMW handling and disposal.

22

Cardiopulmonary Brain Resuscitation (CPBR)

CARDIOPULMONARY BRAIN RESUSCITATION DURING ANAESTHESIA

CPBR is required if cardiac arrest, respiratory arrest or a combination of two occurs. Cardiac arrest or respiratory arrest can occur any where and should be able to resuscitate the victim anywhere without equipments or with equipments according to the situation and availability. CPBR would be required when the **cardiorespiratory arrest occur in the operating room during induction, during surgery or after surgery**.

The main objective of CPBR is to restore oxygen delivery to the brain and other body tissues immediately. It is an acute procedure and should not be delayed. The brain cannot withstand lack of oxygen more than three minutes and the resuscitation should start promptly.

The signs of cardiac arrest are:

1. Absence of pulse (carotid/femoral).
2. Cyanosis or pallor (ash-grey colour).
3. Sudden loss of consciousness in an awake patient.
4. Apnoea or gasping respiration in a spontaneously breathing patient.
5. Dilated pupils.
6. Dark blood on the operation site.

The steps to be followed are:

1. Stop all anaesthetic; give 100% O_2 and continue artificail respiration. Intubate the patient immediately, check for his tracheal tube if intubated.
2. Inform the surgeon and stop the procedure.
3. Call for help.

4. Give a thump on the chest, if no response, start external cardiac compression. Heel of one hand over the other place on the lower third of the sternum. Depress it sharply 4 to 5 cm and release it without taking the hands, at a rate of 100 compressions per minute (Figs 22.1a to c). While external cardiac compression, the elbows of the both hands to be straight.

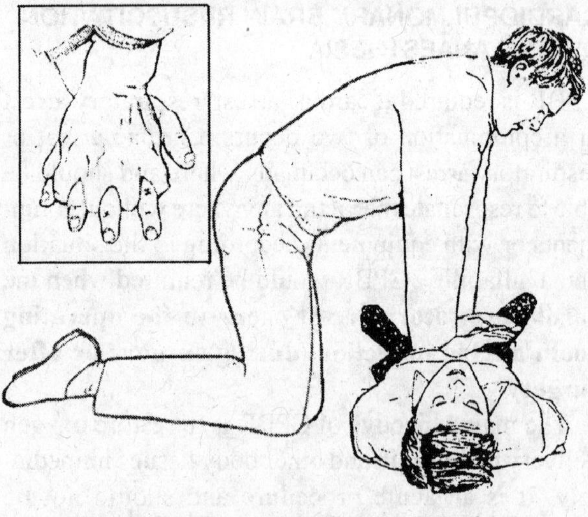

Fig. 22.1a: External cardiac compressions

5. Transfuse fluids if too much blood loss or fluid loss (Crystalloids, colloids, blood, blood products–whichever is available to fill the volume) Exclude the possibility of any concealed bleeding.

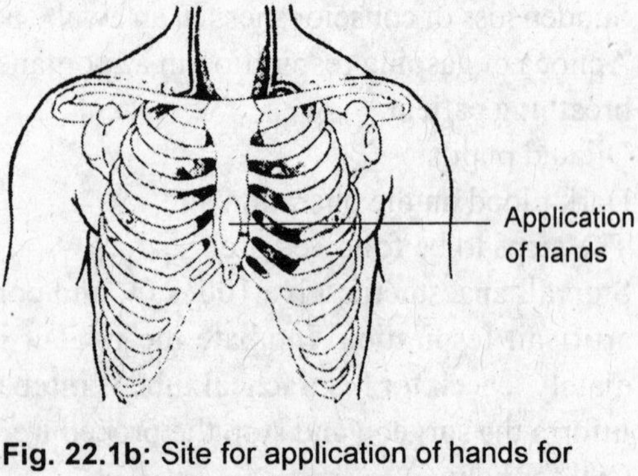

Fig. 22.1b: Site for application of hands for external cardiac compression

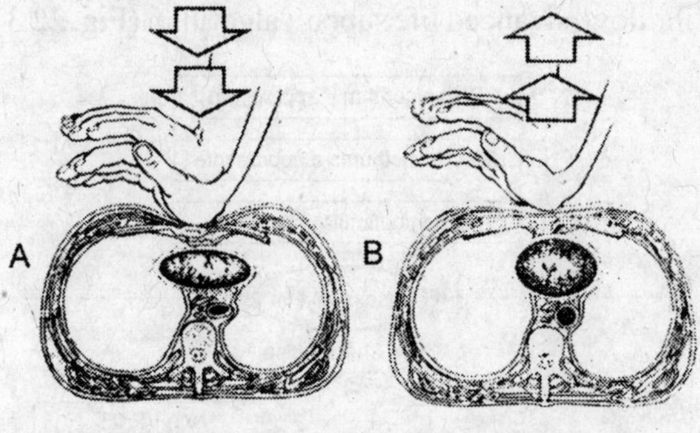

Fig. 22.1c: External cardiac compressions—Lower 1/3 of sternum

6. If cardiac standstill, dilute adrenaline one mgm intravenously or if life line not available, intratracheally and continue external cardiac compression.
7. If ventricular fibrillation, DC shock; charge the machine, apply electrode jelly on the defibrillator (external cardiac compressions) paddles (Fig. 22.2). Place one electrode on the apex and another over the right second sternal border; ask everyone to stay away from the bed and press the paddle button. If not effective increase to more joules and repeat the same.

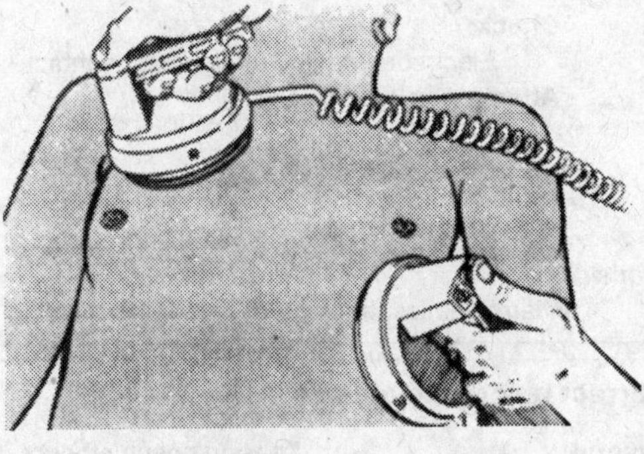

Fig. 22.2: Placement of paddles for external electric defibrillation

8. Assistant should help the anaesthetist in all activities.

9. Follow advanced life support algorithm (Fig. 22.3).

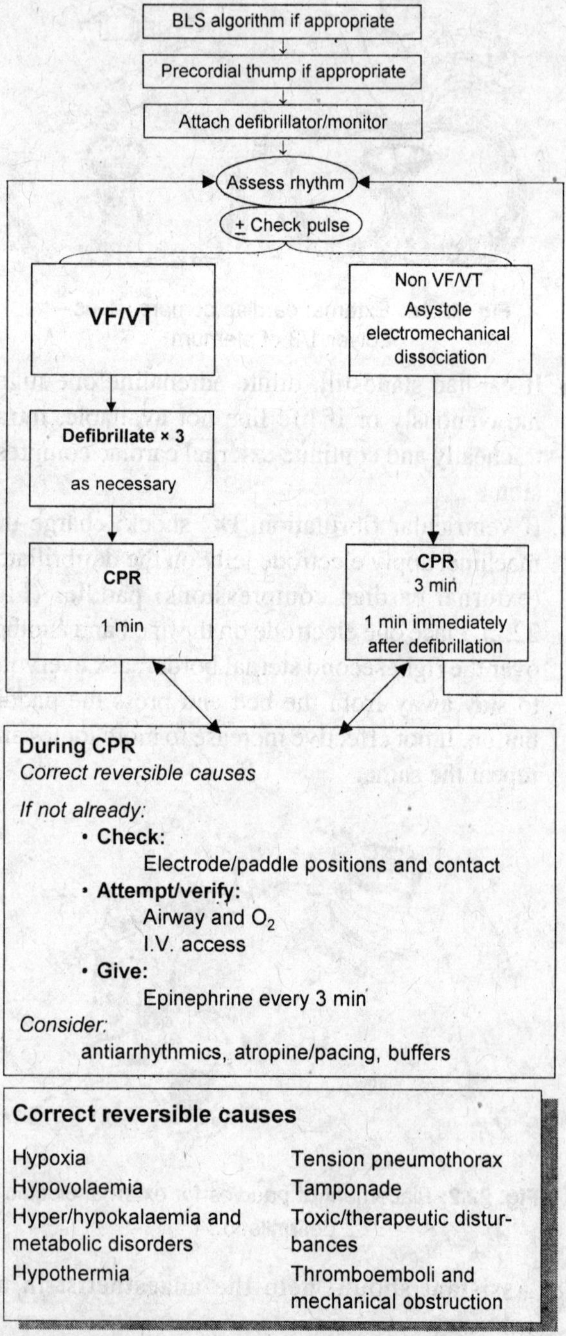

Fig. 22.3: Algorithm: Advanced life support